the guru in you

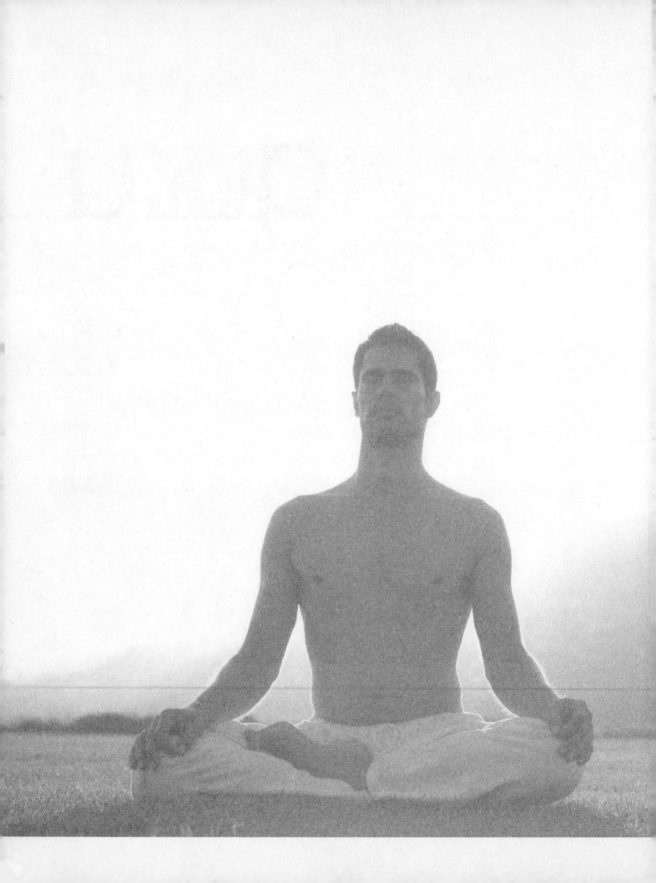

the guru in you

a personalized program for rejuvenating your body and soul

unlock the powers of health and healing within

YOGI CAMERON ALBORZIAN

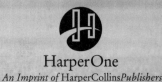

HarperOne
An Imprint of HarperCollinsPublishers

HarperOne

THE GURU IN YOU: *A Personalized Program for Rejuvenating Your Body and Soul.* Copyright © 2011 by Cameron Alborzian. All rights reserved. Printed in the United States of America. No part of this book may be used or reproduced in any manner whatsoever without written permission except in the case of brief quotations embodied in critical articles and reviews. For information address HarperCollins Publishers, 10 East 53rd Street, New York, NY 10022.

HarperCollins books may be purchased for educational, business, or sales promotional use. For information please write: Special Markets Department, HarperCollins Publishers, 10 East 53rd Street, New York, NY 10022.

HarperCollins website: http://www.harpercollins.com

HarperCollins®, ■®, and HarperOne™ are trademarks of HarperCollins Publishers

FIRST EDITION

Library of Congress Cataloging-in-Publication Data is available upon request.

ISBN 978–0–06–189803–7

10 11 12 13 14   RRD(H)   10 9 8 7 6 5 4 3 2 1

For Ron, my mentor and friend,

who put me on the path

contents

contents

viii

introduction

I T WAS TO BE A SHORT WALK after a very long day.

During my second day at Arsha Yoga Vidya Peetam Trust in Coimbatore, India, I had participated in a puja ceremony, taken a yoga posture class, met my guru for the first time, had lunch, attended a lecture on Ayurvedic theory, and observed my guru attend to several patients. I was also still jet-lagged from my flight to India the day before.

"Excuse me, sir?"

I turned around. It was a boy no older than sixteen. He was one of the many teenagers I had encountered who had studied at the center since they were as young as six years old.

"What can I do for you?" I asked.

"What is your good name?"

"Cameron."

"You're from America." It was a statement, not a question. I was the only Westerner at the center.

"Actually, I grew up in Iran and then England, but I have been living in America for a number of years, so sort of."

"That is very good," the boy said. "You have different clothes from us, yes?" He pointed to my simple T-shirt and khakis.

"Yes, very different clothes."

"And different movies?"

"Yes. You have Bollywood, and we have Hollywood."

"Yes! Yes! Holywod. And music? You have different music?" The boy had grown more and more excited with his interrogation. I, however, was remembering my long day and was getting tired.

"Yes. Different music," I said.

"Who do you have for your music?" he asked.

"You mean, what are some of our popular names?"

"Yes! Who do you have?"

I thought for a moment. It was 2003, and I figured at sixteen he would like to hear about the contemporary people. "Well, we have people like Kylie Minogue, Pink, and Eminem. Have you heard of them?"

"No."

"Oh." Perhaps that was too contemporary. "How about something more old-school, like Michael Jackson? Have you heard of him?"

"Yes, not at all."

I considered this as we continued to walk. Then I smiled.

"Have you heard of . . . Madonna?"

"Oh! May-don?" he asked.

"Yes, Madonna, you know, like a virgin."

"No, I've not heard of him."

"Oh. I see. Well, in America, Madonna is a very famous singer, and she puts on huge concerts for thousands of people."

"Wow." The boy's large eyes grew even wider.

"She practices yoga too," I added.

"Really? She doesn't spend money like other famous people?"

"Well, no, she certainly spends money. When I first met her she owned three cars."

"Three cars? Why would somebody have three cars?" he asked.

"To drive them, I suppose."

"That is funny. She can only ever drive one of them at a time."

"Yes, I suppose that is true." We were approaching the apartment complex.

"It sounds like America is a very material place to be."

"Oh, yes, we in the West are living in a material world." I almost groaned to myself.

"She must be very famous if she can afford three cars."

"She's definitely very famous. Some might argue that she's more famous than Jesus Christ."

"Jesus Christ! I've heard of him!"

I laughed. "Of course you have."

As I prepared for bed, I reflected on the coincidence that this boy had used the term *material* to describe America. Along with the different music, movies, and clothes, America and the rural part of India where I was studying couldn't have been more different. I remembered how my own career in fashion not only had earned me money, status, and fame, but it had also led me to appear in the acclaimed "Express Yourself" video starring none other than the Material Girl herself. Going from that life to a three-bedroom apartment in India shared with ten other people showed just how far I had journeyed.

It had been a very long day indeed.

. . .

According to yogic philosophy, time on earth exists in cycles that each span thousands of years. At the beginning of a cycle, the world exists in a denser, more material plane and gradually moves toward a lighter, more awakened realm. Right now, in the twenty-first century, we are at the very beginning of a cycle and therefore are in our densest form. Much as the above story suggests, we really are living in a material world. At this point in the cycle we have a natural affinity for physical appearance, possessions, and decadence. Some might spend their time enjoying their abundance of such things while others spend their time yearning for them. In line with the teachings I have been exposed to, I believe that the many of us who obsess over these things are creating an even denser presence in the world. This presence is furthering our suffering rather than creating a sense of peace and joy. With this book, I aim to teach you as I have been taught. I will show you not only the significance of this suffering but also how to find your way out of the material plane and into joy.

the promise of a better life

Consider two images. The first is a leaf stemming from the branch of a tree. The second is of a person. The leaf is green and vibrant and is absorbing the many rays of light pouring out of the sun. It exists naturally. The person is rushing around trying to achieve things and is struggling with some sort of problem, and as a result this person is slouching and has bags under the eyes. What is significant about these two images is that both of them are common. Many of us wear the obstacles of everyday life as a burden, and this burden manifests as disease and pain in our bodies. We lack sleep, eat foods that tax rather than nurture our bodies, and are susceptible to many ailments that we have accepted as normal. We also, however, see many leaves on many trees that live and thrive exactly as they are intended to—full of vibrancy and energy.

We are intended to live like those leaves. We choose not to.

The work I am presenting to you in this book is based on creating a practice defined by the path of yoga and Ayurveda as set out thousands of years ago. It calls upon all of us to strip away the parts of our lives that tax our bodies and keep us from living in the balanced state that nature originally intended for us. You and I didn't set the rules of nature, but we do have the opportunity to follow them. For thousands of years many generations of people committed themselves to refining this practice, and from their experiences we learn that when we remove inessential parts or habits from our lives, we find our way back to the truest version of ourselves. We create a life for ourselves that is free of disease, sadness, and pain. We understand what contentment is. We understand love. We become as vibrant and joyful as the many leaves that have filled every landscape since the beginning of time.

discovering the guru in you

The word *guru* is a Sanskrit term that means "teacher." This book's title is based on the fact that to truly walk a path that leads to a joyful existence, each of us must find and use tools to strip away inessential layers of our being until we reveal the natural essence of who we are. Consider the act of stripping an old wooden building whose walls have been painted over ten or a dozen times. The paint may be worn or new on the surface, and it may be cracked or smooth. However, if we remove all of the paint, we will discover a natural, unblemished set of boards that radiate the very beauty that earned them a place on the side of the building in the first place. These boards represent what we call our root or our inner guru. The path of yoga and Ayurveda helps us to remove all of the limitations and obstacles that stand in the way of radiating our natural beauty, and when we exist in this natural state, our choices and actions reflect the teachings of this guru—or sacred sense of self. This is not to say, though, that we have no need for a teacher or guidelines such as those outlined in this book. In the beginning we need guidance. It is our responsibility to decide what type of guidance we will pursue.

Many people committed to personal growth begin by reading spiritual books. Reading books and attending seminars and paying for expensive products are all passive behaviors. If you choose a book to help you grow, then that book must also provide specific tools for you to put into practice right away—even before you've finished reading the book. If you don't take time to practice these tools and instead move on to another book or seminar, then you are undermining your chances of ever actually growing out of suffering or understanding why certain experiences keep finding you. The fundamental concept of this book is very simple: the only way out of suffering is to set an intention to change and then practice that change every day.

understanding this book

You may have noticed in the previous section that I described the act of practicing change and therefore used the word *practice* as a verb. Throughout this book, the word *practice* also refers to the series of actions we take to make that change happen. There is a posture practice and a breathing practice. There is a practice of nonviolence and a practice of detachment. We not only can practice something, we can have a practice as well. Posture, breathing, and nonviolence make up a daily routine, and this routine forms a practice. Such a practice is outlined in this book.

The practice in this book is based on teachings that originated in India many centuries ago. However, many of the clients I have worked with often seem intimidated by beginning a practice inspired by ancient teachings. They speak of "all those scary terms" and protest that they're "not flexible enough" to practice yoga postures. The path presented in *The Guru in You* reflects yogic teachings also followed and taught by my guru and his lineage, and the fundamental concept of these teachings is that a beneficial yoga and Ayurveda practice is much simpler than it's often made out to be. These practices are intended to help us access our true selves, not scare us out of wanting to do the necessary work. The most challenging aspect of this practice isn't learning complicated terms and mastering difficult yoga postures; instead, it is making this type of practice a priority and sustaining our commitment to it. With the exception of a few terms like *guru* and *yoga*, I have refrained from using Sanskrit words to describe these practices. Many of the exercises that I suggest have been designed to fit into your everyday life, such as when you go to lunch with a friend or are watching a football game. As you explore these practices, it will be your responsibility to observe which layers of your life are useful to you and which are not.

The Guru in You is divided into three parts. The first part, "The Path," introduces the concepts behind this practice as it relates to the material world and the first steps for committing yourself to the pursuit of a fully realized life of joy and peace.

The second part, "Foundation," outlines three basic behaviors to modify if you want to establish a sound basis for your practice that will support long-term change. While physical practices like posture and breathing are a very important part of this path, these practices need to be grounded by a commitment to the path in the form of conscious living. The tools provided in this part center on abstaining from certain behaviors as dictated not just by yogic tradition but by other traditions as well (the Ten Commandments, the Quran, the Torah, and so forth). Though yoga is not a religion, as the oldest spiritual path, all other traditions have a basis in its philosophies and concepts.

The third part, "Expression," presents a series of practices that many of us commonly associate with yoga, such as postures and breathing exercises. We consider these tools an expression of our practice because they are a more outward and mechanical component of the path than the foundational tools outlined in the second part.

The word *yoga* is derived from the Sanskrit word *yuj*, which means to yoke or join. The fourth and final part, "Union," consists of one chapter that will help you to yoke the many tools outlined in this book into one cohesive practice.

Perhaps the most important thing for you to know before you begin this journey is that you are not alone on your quest. In this book I include stories from my own life that show my transition from the fashion industry into a life committed to the practice and teaching of yoga and Ayurveda. These stories illustrate the very concepts that will help you to find the guru in you. In presenting these practices, I also include a variety of stories from the work I have done with my many different clients as well as the exercises that form the foundation of this practice. My work often includes staying with a client anywhere from a day to a week, depending on their condition. I move in all of my Ayurvedic equipment, which includes herbs, a treatment aparatus, medicated oils, and medicines. I stay until the root cause of the disease or ailment has been identified and the person is better. The methods in *The Guru in You* reflect the processes I employ when working with my clients and can be used for your personal application.

I offer the tools in this book not with the goal of dictating the only way to create real and significant change in your life, but rather to show you a specific process that has been of value to many people over thousands of years. There are many different paths to self-realization, and it can often seem daunting to find your own way. If you do choose to use the tools introduced in this book over the course of your life, then you will create change. If you use a different set of tools, then you will also create change. The only way to find your own path, however, is to begin with something and stick to it over the course of years. Discovering your inner guru begins with practicing change, and when you do so you will begin to free yourself of the burdens centered on living in the material world. When you do this, you will realize the greatest, most inspired version of yourself.

For what, in the end, is more important than joy?

the path

the material world

1

R ON PICKED UP THE STATUETTE from the table. It was an
arrangement of triangular shapes sculpted over a simple marble base,
and it said, "Cameron Alborzian— Best Male Model, The Fashion
Industry Awards, 1993." We were seated at a table along the dance
floor in the basement level of the Les Bain Douche nightclub in Paris.

"Explain to me," Ron said, "why we came here to get this today."

I shrugged. "They said they were holding it here for me. And you looked
like you could use a night out anyway, mate."

"I know they were holding it here for you, but that was because you
didn't get it when they presented it to you."

"Right," I said.

"At the awards ceremony."

"Yes."

"Held here in this very room."

I nodded.

"Last night."

I looked around the room. Indeed, the way it was currently set up was
a stark contrast to how it must have looked the previous night with tables
filling the room and a podium up onstage for the French fashion industry's first awards ceremony. Tonight the dance floor was open, and the
stage looked ready for a musical act—though we were only listening to
background music at the moment.

Ron was my best friend, and he and I liked going to Les Bain Douche, along with the rest of the trend-loving residents of Paris. I was certainly fond of being able to walk up to the most famous club in the city and be let right in, though this was only one of many perks of being in the business I was in.

"He gets an award for being the best model in the business—"

"The best *male* model."

"Fine. You and Christy Turlington could form a club. And he doesn't even care enough to show up at the club on the actual night the awards ceremony takes place."

I laughed at my friend. He had been a model himself when he was younger and had hung out with folks like Grace Jones and Keith Haring during his own career in the business. He never seemed moved to comment one way or the other on the work I did, but for whatever reason he wanted to discuss the awards ceremony.

"So are you going for another award for Most Detached Model or something?"

I shrugged. Ron just shook his head.

"What do you want me to say?" I asked.

"Nothing, Cameron. Just promise you'll remember who your friends are when you've taken over the—"

"Shhh," I said. "I think something's about to happen."

The doors had closed and the lights gone down. We didn't know if anyone was playing that night, so we were as surprised as everyone else when none other than The Artist Formerly Known as Prince came on the stage.

Life in fashion certainly kept things interesting.

. . .

Because I worked in the fashion business, most of my friends came from one entertainment industry or another. Ron, however, was a different story. I had met him at the gym when two of my fashion buddies, Joey and Paul, and I were doing bad Rocky impressions among the free weights ("Just one more rep, Rock-o!"). I saw Ron from across the room, and somehow we found ourselves talking as if we had always known each other. On the surface we may have seemed an odd couple—I was a nineteen-year-old straight man just starting out in life, and he was a middle-aged gay former model squeaking by in a shabby sublet apartment—but we became friends all the same. We spent a lot of time together. Being diagnosed with HIV in 1985, however, changed much of how Ron lived his life, so when we became friends in 1986, I learned to know a person with a much different perspective than my own. Still, he enjoyed his fair share of gossip about things happening at fashion industry awards shows.

None of our differences—nor the eyebrow raising I received from my friends—dampened the closeness I felt to Ron. He was my most intimate confidant as I continued to rise through the ranks of the fashion industry, working for designers like Versace, Chanel, and Valentino. He saw me through several relationships, a troubled marriage, and the birth of my daughter.

Around the time I was busy not attending awards shows, I decided to buy an apartment in Paris for Ron to live in. I rented another home in New York City, which I lived in for much of the year, but when I was in Paris I lived in this other apartment with Ron. By 1997 I had worked with most of the top designers in fashion and had traveled much of the world meeting all kinds of people. On a warm fall day in Paris, my agency sent me to a casting for a catalog shoot. At the time I was doing magazine campaigns, but this client had requested I come by for consideration. I walked into the lobby of the client's studio, which was filled with over a dozen men. One man who seemed to be in his early forties turned to me as I took a seat near the door.

"Cameron," he said. "Loved the Levi's campaign you did a couple of years back."

"Well, thank you," I said. I recognized the man from various shoots, but I didn't know his name.

"And what was Elton John like to work with in that video? What was the name of that song again?"

"Working with him was fine. The song was called 'Something About the Way You Look Tonight.'"

He furrowed his brow for a moment.

"What are you doing here?" he asked. "Going for the money?"

"What do you mean?"

"Well, I never see you in any catalogs, just the high-fashion magazines. None of us really do catalog shoots until we have to, do we?" He gestured around the room.

I looked too. Most of the men were, in fact, older, sustaining the latter parts of their careers by doing catalog gigs. Catalogs paid okay, but nothing compared to the Versaces and Chanels of the world. When I looked back at the man, his brow was still furrowed, and his eyes never met mine again.

On my way home I considered our conversation. What struck me was not that he assumed his work as a middle-aged model would be based mostly on catalogs, but that he seemed so profoundly dissatisfied with it. He couldn't imagine why a model still in his thirties and in the prime of his career would even consider a catalog gig. His furrowed brow painted a picture of what was to come, and it was not an attractive view.

"What do you think of this picture?" Ron asked. I had arrived home to find him standing among several small boxes. His illness was showing its effects: much of his hair had fallen out since we had first met, and his clothes no longer fit. He was losing weight.

"That's your Keith Haring drawing, right?" Haring had given it to Ron only a couple of years before his death in 1990.

"Yeah. Peter would like it, wouldn't he?" He put the drawing neatly in a box labeled *P*.

"I'm sorry?" I asked, distracted.

"I'm giving the drawing to Peter. My pic with Grace Jones too."

These were some of Ron's most prized possessions, and Peter was a friend of his. I didn't understand. I watched as he took some raw emeralds and sapphires and placed them in a different box labeled *S*. The gems must have been worth several thousand dollars.

"This box is for Samir," he said. Samir was a friend of his who collected artifacts. Along with the stones, he filled Samir's box with various statues from different places around the world.

"Ron, why—?"

"I don't have any need for them anymore, Cameron."

I thought about the way the model at the casting had lamented his life in catalogs. The man's eyes betrayed his despair at having no options beyond fading into a secondary career in fashion. The man seemed to be in perfect health, but like Ron, he also seemed to be wasting away. Unlike this other man, however, when Ron said that he didn't have any need for the objects, his eyes showed nothing of despair.

Even though he was ill, his eyes were filled with life.

the material world

Because of my status in the fashion industry, the doors to clubs were always open, I was getting the most desirable jobs, I had the nicest clothes, I was able to afford a part-time home in Paris while paying for my best friend to live there year-round, and even had worked with Madonna quite literally in her "material world." By many people's standards, there was little else I could want in life. At no point during that period of my life, however, did I feel the lightness that I perceived in Ron when he was freeing himself of his more cherished possessions.

Many of us either fill our lives with material goods and live a lavish lifestyle or else aspire to do so, pursuing more money and more extravagant experiences. We crave certain foods, value decadence and luxury as the good life, envy and follow physically beautiful people in the fashion and entertainment industries, and fill our homes with souvenirs from the past. During my studies in India and throughout the world, I learned that the many of us who obsess over these things are creating an even denser attachment to the world. It is the goal of this chapter to teach you how to become more aware of your heaviness in the actual, material world. I will show how this attachment does not create a sense of contentment and joy but instead furthers suffering.

I also have very good news. In the introduction, I mentioned that Indian philosophy considers time on earth to exist in cycles. These cycles are known as *yugas,* and each is thought to span many years. Though this concept has been open to various interpretations, the general agreement is that right now in the twenty-first century we are in this denser, more material form and are about to pursue our collective awakening. At this point in the cycle we have a natural affinity for physical appearance, possessions, and decadence. Each one of us on earth is subject to this material affinity, and every person is conspiring with every other person to ensure that we all stay firmly rooted in this plane. We've added layer after layer of material dependence, and in some ways we're perpetuating our state. How is any of this good news? It's very simple: whatever unhappiness or dissatisfaction has brought you to this book is a product of this cycle and is to be expected.

More good news is that before any of these material layers added themselves to our existence, each of us began life in a state of joy. With practice, we can strip away those layers and fully realize this joy once more.

the material world in our everyday lives

It is easy to see material abundance all around us. People live in enormous homes, eat at fancy restaurants, wear designer clothes, decorate themselves with opulent jewels, and drive enormous cars that burn up a gallon of gas for every ten miles driven. Luxury and decadence are the most obvious forms of the material plane, and whether we live such a lifestyle or merely covet it—and during a recession most people only covet it—most of us can on some level relate to feeling that this way of life is ideal.

Let us reflect, though, on the story that began this chapter. My own station in the fashion industry gave me the unqualified opportunity to enjoy being catered to and to own more than one home. I had the means to travel wherever I wanted and go without work for weeks at a time when I felt like it. However, it was not adding more and more of these luxuries but instead removing them that led Ron's eyes to shine with happiness and peace—even if for only a moment.

MONEY

We often assign the term *materialistic* to someone who puts a tremendous value on money and expensive things. A ring is only a good ring if it is very expensive. A work of art is valuable not because of the emotional reaction it creates in the viewer but because of how much money it is worth. A car is not just a mode of transporting oneself from point A to point B but also a statement of one's economic status. While it may be easy to label people who think this way as materialistic, most of us in fact tend to place more value on objects and experiences that cost more money.

Assigning value to something through a dollar amount keeps one entrenched in the material world. Pursuing a more awakened realm does not necessarily mean never valuing anything that costs money, but it does promote a desire to value quality goods and experiences over expensive ones. The next time you're presented with the option of going to two restaurants—one of which is a modest place known for particularly tasty food and the other an upscale and expensive restaurant known only for being upscale and expensive—ask yourself whether you value a quality experience or merely an expensive one.

POSSESSIONS

Many of us define our self-worth by our material possessions. We worship and crave the things humans produce instead of what is created by nature. Even if we aren't coveting the most expensive handbags and the biggest houses, most of us can relate to a desire to have objects in our lives. They can be objects with significant commercial value, like designer clothes or jewelry, or objects with greater sentimental value, like a gift someone gave us or an important photograph. While we think that having these things is creating happiness in our lives, we're actually responding to an idea or memory that we associate with them. You might care deeply for a photograph because it was the last one you had taken with your mother before she passed away, but the existence of the photograph is not what creates your love for her. Your memories are what create that feeling, and having the photograph isn't necessary to validate the affection you feel for her. If an accident were to happen that destroyed that photograph, you would have an opportunity to celebrate your mother's life by expressing that affection toward another or telling her story to someone who never knew her.

FOOD

If we're to pursue a lighter, more awakened realm in our lives, then rich, heavy foods will impede that pursuit. They are, of course, hard to resist, as few things seem more satisfying than a moist piece of cake or a greasy slice of pizza. It may seem obvious, but dense foods keep us in a denser state of being and will often lead to getting an upset stomach or experiencing a midafternoon slump or some other form of mild suffering. I'm always amused by how much my friends and family eat on a holiday like Thanksgiving, spending the rest of the day complaining about how bloated they feel and how they ate too much.

Eating these kinds of foods in great abundance and on a regular basis may seem satisfying at the time, but they offer little help in your pursuit of greater joy. Later in the book we'll explore food through the lens of the ancient system of Ayurveda, which will give guidelines on how to pursue better eating habits.

give a prized object away

Many of us associate a spiritual practice with lots of breathing techniques and the contemplation of higher forms of living. There are also very simple ways to begin practicing awareness in our day-to-day lives. It's important to remember, though, that just because an exercise is simple doesn't mean that it's easy.

One of the ways we are bound to the material world is by collecting artifacts that we value from our past, such as Ron's drawings and precious gems. This first exercise to become more aware of the material world is to give one of your own artifacts away. This can be a trinket someone special gave you for your birthday, a medal you were given to recognize your service to an organization, or even something of significant commercial value, like a piece of jewelry or autographed sporting goods memorabilia. By giving an important and valued possession away, you're creating an opportunity to reflect on how the absence of that object makes you feel.

Observe how you feel immediately after giving away the object.

If you feel a lightness similar to what I observed in Ron, then you probably didn't need the object cluttering up your life in the first place. Try giving something else away that may challenge you a bit more.

If you feel a sense of loss after giving it away, then this is where the real work of observing yourself in this practice begins. If you were to give away your deceased grandmother's necklace and it was the only object you had to remind you of her, this is an

SUCCESS

Anyone in a corporate or institutional work environment can relate to the prospect of success as defined by upward mobility. Many of us want to be what we call successful, and we often value our lives by the extent to which we attain that success. Setting a goal that we would like to achieve and then working toward that goal can certainly benefit our temporary happiness, as long as we find the results of that work to our liking. But rather than focus our attention on a long-lasting and rooted joy, many of us define our sense of worth by the extent to which we've attained corporate, institutional, or personal success. This disturbs our balance and creates problems for us.

opportunity to invest your energy instead in celebrating the time you had with her.

If you feel crippled by the absence of this object and are unable to think of anything else, then try to make light of the situation. For example, ask the person you gave it to for visiting rights. Like I said, this exercise is simple enough to execute, but if we assign a tremendous amount of value to an object, it can be very difficult to give it away.

If the object was given to you by someone who is still very much a part of your life, then by all means talk with this person first and explain why giving the object away indicates only your own desire for growth and is not in any way a negative comment on your feelings for them. You might even suggest that your friend try giving something away as well—though by this point it may be you!

When you feel you have resolved any feelings of loss over the object, consider giving something else away. Continue to observe how no longer having these objects makes you feel.

You may find that it is not too challenging to give away a possession to a loved one. If this is the case, then try giving a prized possession to someone you find it difficult to like or someone you dislike outright. This will be a good release for you and for the other person.

As I said before, this exercise may be simple, but it's also very ambitious. Begin with smaller objects, and work your way up from there. The more awareness you bring to this experience, the less you'll be controlled by your emotions and the greater your potential is for growth. The more our emotions rule us, the further the truth is from our sight.

APPEARANCE

Having been in the fashion business for over ten years, I was exposed to many people who valued outer beauty as a defining aspect of a person's worth. The entire industry of fashion grows from the idea that we must base our value as people on our appearance and that the folks walking the runways and posing in pictures have the tools to build that value in ourselves. The advertising industry takes a similar tack, as the success of their business stems from selling the public on the idea that self-worth can be had only by using more products and pampering services. As I'm sure you can imagine, defining our worth in such a way works against our happiness, as it is not our outer beauty but our inner beauty that needs to be cultivated over the course of our lives.

This idea is so common that it is often expressed in clichés: "Beauty is in the eye of the beholder," "Don't judge a book by its cover," and so forth. But this in no way diminishes the importance of the message: our joy is fully realized by celebrating our inner beauty as human beings. Many of the practices outlined in this book will help you value inner beauty within yourself and those around you.

FITNESS

Many people want to be physically fit, but they make it their goal to have the right butt, abs, and legs rather than to simply be healthy. There are even some people who become addicted to an idea of physical fitness to the point that they can barely function if they don't spend part of each day running on the treadmill, using the weight machine, or weighing themselves on the scale. When we regard fitness in the context of freeing ourselves from the material world, we work toward valuing physical movement and exercise as a way to foster a sense of balance and peace in our bodies and minds. While this may include having a regular exercise routine to maintain a healthy flow of energy, it certainly doesn't include taxing our bodies to the point of creating soreness, anxiety, and even injury. The chapter on yoga postures later in this book will explain this idea in greater detail.

FAMILY

You may be asking, Oh, no, is he going to say there's something wrong with having a family? No, of course I'm not going to say this. The potential problem arises not in having a family but in how we define ourselves in relation to family. Many people feel their lives will have no meaning if they don't have children or aren't surrounded by a large family. I've heard many stories from childless, middle-aged clients who describe other people challenging them and even ostracizing them because they chose not to have children. These confrontational or fearful people decided that a person's life, to be valuable, must include children. In this practice we are leaving behind limited perceptions like this. When we pursue an awakening of our purpose and joy, we do so with the understanding that this joy can grow with as many or as few people as we find enrich our lives.

the weight of the material world

A question worth asking, though, is: Why should it be necessary to remove ourselves from a material existence? Wouldn't it be easier to go along as we always did, relishing the richness of an abundant and expensive existence? My response to this is the story of my client Michael.

Michael worked as a manager and editor of national magazines. He carried the responsibility for the success and prosperity of several publications, and he led several thousand employees toward commercial success year after year. He traveled the world, met great people, owned four homes, and earned the salary to pay for it all. You might consider him a model of success because he lived the life that many of us only dream of.

When he came to me, Michael complained of allergies and digestion issues, and he didn't sleep well. His pursuit of success and corporate prosperity was relentless. Though he tempered himself in most situations, he sometimes felt paranoid that those working for him were trying to undermine his authority, such as trying to make him look bad in front of his own boss so that they could steal his job. He found that if he was unable to control other people as he worked to get what he wanted, he would burst like an angry volcano. This would cause him to feel even worse about himself afterward, and his allergic and digestive issues would worsen. When he came to me, he felt that his position at his company was in jeopardy, for he was beginning to get a reputation for being abusive and impossible to work with. He was desperate for change.

Michael is a perfect example of a person entrenched in the confines of the material world. He based much of his self-worth on how successfully and expensively he lived his life, as his greatest source of stress stemmed from not being able to succeed and get what he wanted. Essentially, the material world was growing in Michael like a cyst. To counter this reality, I gave his lifestyle an overhaul. He liked eating rich and creamy foods, so I switched him to fruits, vegetables, whole grains, and light forms of foods that were easy to digest. His eruptive nature was based in part on his inclination to hold his breath, so I had him practice breathing exercises to encourage a more even-tempered disposition. Over time we worked together to bring balance to his life, and as he grew to observe himself in situations that had previously caused conflicts, he was able to separate himself from his obsession with becoming more successful. While he still worked hard, his inclination to lose his temper no longer seemed necessary. Michael learned to control himself and not others.

Six months later Michael was still at his job and still very successful, but he was no longer the least bit fearful of his station there. His motivation was pleasure in his work rather than fear. His employees seemed happy and so did he. He had begun the process of freeing himself of the material world, even though he still participated in it through taking responsibility for his job and meeting financial obligations. While each of us has an opportunity to begin freeing ourselves of this denser state of being, we will also need to ground our pursuit of freedom by satisfying other needs, as Michael did by continuing to prosper in his job. Observing ourselves in this balancing act forms a major component of our practice.

As I stated earlier, the goal of this chapter is to teach you to become more aware of your place in the material world, and the chapters that follow will show you how to develop a practice that will help you liberate yourself from this reality. As you continue on with your practice, you'll begin to learn how significant your connection to the material world really is.

. . .

Returning to my original story, I helped Ron pack up several more boxes of his possessions that day. True to his word, he gave everything away. This made a significant impression on me.

I might have been working for major fashion clients, had a wardrobe filled with some of the finest garments, and found success in some music videos, but nothing about my life inspired the sense of freedom and joy that emanated from Ron when he decided to free himself of all his unnec-

sit before you veg

If you're like almost everyone I know, your first impulse when you get home from a long day at work or a busy day running errands is to grab a bag of chips, a beer, or some kind of snack, sprawl out on the couch, and watch TV for four hours before going to bed. You may have had a conflict with a co-worker or felt overwhelmed by the long lines at the supermarket, and with so much drudgery and frustration, the last thing you want to do is something productive—like reading to your kids, paying your bills, or finishing certain chores.

This makes perfect sense. When we feel overwhelmed by the dense energy that fills our hectic lives, we think we need to neutralize the bad heaviness with things that supposedly make us feel good: eating sweet and oily foods, watching aimless television programs, and finding the most horizontal position we can for our bodies to experience weightlessness. While these may seem satisfying at the moment, they add heaviness to our material bodies, which burdens us and keeps us further entrenched in our own suffering.

This exercise calls upon you to create a short sitting practice for yourself when you feel you're ready to submit to your end-of-day impulses or even sleepiness at the office. It is designed to foster alertness, which will counter the inevitable lethargy of a taxing day. When you're done with work or errands or have finished your dinner, find somewhere quiet in your home or office to sit in a basic cross-legged position. This can be in the middle of the floor, against a wall, or even on a chair with your feet on the ground if you find significant discomfort in sitting with crossed legs. Close your eyes, and take long and slow breaths. Breathe in through your nose for a count of three, and then breathe out through your nose for a count of six. Repeat this thirty times or however many times you feel comfortable with. The breathing will deliver more oxygen to your entire body, which will stimulate cellular activity in the brain and calm the nerves.

In later chapters you will learn more about breathing, sitting, and other elements of this exercise, but for now consider the following points:

- As this exercise is designed to foster alertness, it is important to have an erect spine. If sitting cross-legged makes your shoulders slump forward and your lower back sink, sit on a couple of folded blankets or a yoga block to raise your pelvis. This will help to properly align your spine.

- If breathing in and out through your nose is difficult for you, try breathing in through your nose and then out through your mouth.

Once you've completed the breathing, sit for a moment and observe how you feel about vegging out as opposed to doing something you've been putting off. Do you want to spend the whole evening watching TV (the TV eventually watches you), or do you want to watch only one of the four shows? Do you want to eat those chips (which eventually become you), or are you willing to try a piece of fruit, sip some herbal tea, or not consume anything at all? A great first step in becoming more aware of your place in this material world is to challenge yourself to crave a lighter energy, and this awareness can begin with the heaviest hours of your day.

essary possessions. Ron's condition became terminal and he was left with only a couple of years to live, but during that time he was filled with more life than anyone I had ever known. Though I would eventually adjust my own life to fall more in line with Ron's actions, it would be several more years before I made the decision to change my role in the material world forever.

fill in the blank

Just like a sentence with a missing word has no meaning, a practice without action has no beginning. Each chapter of this book will end with a reminder to try one or more of its exercises as part of this beginning. In putting down this book and practicing, you are writing your own conclusion to this chapter and its practices; you are filling in the blank.

The following chapter will teach you the importance of setting an intention. Before learning how this will help you to strengthen your commitment to a life of practice, experiment with building your awareness by sitting for five or ten minutes and giving one of your prized objects away.

setting your intention

2

the first step toward happiness

"CAMERON."

"Yes, Ron."

"I'd like to talk to you about something."

I looked at my friend. "We're already talking, aren't we?"

Ron didn't acknowledge my smart remark and instead said nothing for several moments. He seemed to be brooding over something.

We were taking one of our standard long walks from our flat to the 10th arrondissement of Paris to go to an organic café that served a mushroom and cheese tart we had grown to crave. It wasn't uncommon for us to make the hour-long trek or to walk for even an hour and a half to go to the only health food store in the whole northern half of the city. It was, after all, only 1999, just before the natural foods craze that exploded in the following years. This didn't stop Ron, however, from riding the fashion train of previous decades. That day he was sporting a green jumpsuit and a baseball hat, which he claimed kept him comfortable when restraining Sacchi, our shar-pei/Rhodesian ridgeback mix, from chasing other dogs.

"Cameron, I would like for you to be happy," Ron said.

"What makes you think I'm not happy?" I asked.

"You left the fashion business, what, about a year ago, right?"

I did the math. It had indeed been about a year since I had traveled to South Africa with Kate Moss and some other members of the industry to meet Nelson Mandela for a charity event. That had represented the end of my career, though only because the trip had coincided with my realization that the only work available to me as I progressed through my thirties would be catalog jobs. I realized I had achieved all I wanted in the fashion business by working with the most talented and creative people in the industry. As great as it was working with the best, I no longer felt challenged by the work nor gratified by the fashion rush. In the past year I had partnered with a woman to run a restaurant in New York City and was developing a perfume line as well.

"Yeah, it's been about a year, I guess."

"And do you think you're happy?"

"Well, the restaurant is doing very well. It's gotten a lot of press, and my partner doesn't even seem to need me in New York all that much."

"I know, but that's the restaurant, not you." He paused again. "What do you think all of those spiritual books and lessons we've been sharing over the years have been teaching?"

"They've said all sorts of things," I replied, not knowing where he was going with this. Ron had been studying these books for over ten years and sharing them with me since shortly after we became friends.

"Yes, but regardless of the specific things they say, they've all pretty much pointed to the same basic lesson, wouldn't you say?"

I considered this. We had started heading south on Quai de Jemmapes, along one of the city's many canals. Sacchi took note of a German shepherd across the way, but just as Ron had begun to slow down in his later years, Sacchi disregarded the dog a moment later.

"I suppose," I said, "that they all speak to finding our purpose."

"Right," he said. "And where do they teach us to look for this purpose?"

"In the cash registers of all of the restaurants we own." I laughed. He didn't.

"Cameron, you have an ex-wife who can barely spend ten minutes in the room with you without becoming angry, you flit around from one meaningless relationship to another, and while your businesses may be doing all right, you don't seem to be enjoying the work very much."

I said nothing.

"Your life's a mess. Don't you want to be a good influence on your daughter? Don't you want to be there for your friends?"

"You know the answer to that," I said.

"Yes, I do. Do you?"

I was a little taken aback by this interrogation. We had had many talks during these long walks, and many of them were quite serious. He had never, however, taken me to task like this. Still, I had to admit that while I had read a lot of these spiritual books about finding one's purpose and happiness, I hadn't done much more than go on the occasional yoga retreat and take a few self-help workshops conducted by people like Gurumayi or the people at the Satchidananda Ashram. Ron, by contrast, had gone completely organic in his eating and lived each day with a proenvironment agenda before it was fashionable to go green. I had watched him give away most of his possessions. It was a testament to his daily practice that he not only had survived with HIV for years without any modern medicine, but he was lighter, happier, and more at peace than anyone I had ever known.

Certainly more at peace than anyone I knew in the fashion or restaurant businesses.

"You have so many opportunities that you aren't pursuing," he continued. "And I'm not talking about financial opportunities—"

"I know what you're talking about, Ron."

We had arrived at the café. The small room was filled with the smell of pastries and tarts. In front was a display of postcards from across the world sent by customers of the café. The elderly woman who ran the café wore a smile that took over her entire face. When we walked in she lovingly carried on in French about how pleased she was to have us back. After she gave us both a hug, she knelt down to greet Sacchi, who was always allowed to lie under our table.

After we had ordered our cheese and mushroom tarts, we took a seat near the window. It was a comment on how intent Ron was in having this conversation that he didn't stop to look at the postcards, which he had a habit of doing whenever we came.

"It doesn't matter what you do, Cameron, or how much money you're making. Every one of those teachings says that the only place you can find your happiness is within yourself."

The woman had started wiping down a nearby table.

"You saw her face when we came in," he said. "I just want that for you."

Ron's condition remained stable for a number of months following that day, but by the middle of 2000 his health had taken a turn for the worse. In the summer he had a sense that his time was about up, as not even living his lifestyle was going to save him from the virus. He decided that he wanted to give up eating and to spend his remaining time on his own so he would have an opportunity to reflect.

It was a choice that many people around him found difficult to understand. My instructions when I met his friends at the front door of our building were to turn them away. It had nothing to do with his not having affection for them, for he loved his friends very much. He just knew that, as older members of the gay community who had lost many to the disease, they would be bringing their fear into the home. They would be disrupting his desire to let go of his physical body and die in peace.

A couple of weeks after Ron had stopped eating, I needed to leave Paris to pick up my daughter from her mom's in New York City and bring her to England to begin school near where my parents lived. I knew that Ron's time was running out, so I promised him that I would be back within three days.

"Take care of yourself," he said.

I was emerging from the subway on my way to my ex-wife's apartment in Brooklyn when I got the call.

"Cameron." It was Robert, a dancer friend of Ron's who had been one of the people trying to gain entrance to the flat.

"Cameron, Ron's gone."

"He is," I said.

"Yes, he's gone. He died while the doctors were hooking him up to the machines—"

"Doctors?"

"Yes, the doctors—"

"What doctors, Robert?"

"What doctors? The doctors at the hospital. It's because he had been starving himself for weeks—"

"Why was he at the hospital, Robert?"

"I took him there."

"You took him—"

"Ron wanted to be taken to the hospital."

"I think Ron wanted to do what he wanted to do."

"No, he wanted to be taken to the—Cameron, he was dying. I don't understand how you could let him do this to himself. I don't understand why he wouldn't want to live. Why wouldn't he want to live? Why would he do something like this?"

I didn't say anything.

"Cameron?"

"Yes, Robert."

"Why did he do this?"

At this point in the conversation, I might have yelled at Robert and told him that all that Ron wanted was to die in peace and that Robert had taken that away from him. I could have told him that Ron was ready to leave his body and didn't require a doctor. Robert was a few years older than me; he, like Ron, was HIV-positive and was exhibiting all of the fears that Ron had been so carefully removing himself from when he sequestered himself in our flat. I could have told Robert that he was wrong to do what he did. Thankfully, at that moment I wasn't tempted to say any of that.

"Ron's passing is nothing for us to be afraid of, Robert."

Robert said little else. He hung up. We never spoke again.

Many people on a spiritual path regard the passing of a loved one as a cause, not of mourning, but of celebration. I was no exception. I was in no position to bear Robert or any of his other friends any ill will, for they simply hadn't freed themselves of their fears as Ron had.

In the weeks and months that followed Ron's death, I reflected a great deal on how he lived and what he wanted. While he had been denied the right to die on his own terms, getting HIV all of those years ago had taught him how important it was to let go of everything—including the physical place and the specific circumstances through which he died. In observing his passing, I realized that more than any of the gurus or prominent mind-body-spirit figures from whom I might have taken a seminar or workshop, Ron had been my mentor. He not only had wanted happiness and peace for me, but he also had shown through example that it wasn't enough simply to read a lot of books and go to the occasional ashram or seminar. I needed to take the concepts and apply them every day of my life. It was the difference between thinking about theories of better living and actually practicing them.

. . .

I held the certificate in my hand. It was early 2003, and I had just completed a teacher training at Integral Yoga in New York City's Greenwich Village. I had also completed a reflexology course at the Open Center several weeks prior. The yoga training had been filled with an interesting variety of people who, when they weren't in class, worked as everything from schoolteachers to musicians. The training had lasted six months, and it had given us a body of knowledge about how to practice several dozen postures and a variety of breathing exercises.

As I looked at the certificate that declared me now to be a yoga teacher, I considered how reluctant I was to study with any of those who also held these certificates in their hands. I had no qualms about the excellence of their work or the strength of the program that had prepared us all to be yoga teachers. I simply felt that six months was not enough time for anyone to learn how to teach something that took yogis in India decades to master. It definitely wasn't long enough for me.

When I was completely honest with myself, I had to admit that I had signed up for the various trainings I had just completed merely because I couldn't think of anything else to do. I knew that I wanted to immerse myself in some sort of spiritual practice, as Ron's example had made such a profound impact on me. Yet while I did do some teaching over the next couple of months, I felt somewhat aimless in my pursuits. I began researching other programs in New York and other parts of the United States, but most of them lasted six months or less, much like the program I had just finished. I wanted something more.

I had heard of Ayurveda from people like Deepak Chopra, but I knew little about it. Later in 2003 I discovered that while a yoga practice trains the mind, an Ayurveda lifestyle trains the body. By using both in a complementary and informed way, a person has the opportunity to fully realize a practice of health, purpose, and of course happiness. But there was a great deal of information to learn. Feeling a need for complete immersion in an educational setting, I headed off to India.

It was finally time for me to listen to my mentor's advice.

what is an intention?

We often hear the word *intention* used in our day-to-day lives. When a well-meaning person says something inappropriate without knowing it, others might forgive the faux pas because the person has good intentions. People responsible for the Holocaust, the World Trade Center attacks, and the AIG financial crisis are regarded as having bad intentions.

Your intention, as it relates to the practice of finding the guru in you, is the reason you want to accomplish a goal that you have set for yourself. What would happen if you were working at a company and your supervisor asked you to complete a project but didn't tell you why it needed to be done? You would probably be able to complete the project, but your commitment, focus, and even competence might suffer. Obstacles would become more difficult to overcome, and you wouldn't feel as satisfied upon completing your task. The same is true for the practice outlined in this book. I could give you an eating plan to follow, a series of exercises to practice, and a comprehensive formula for change, and you could probably eat a few different foods and try out a few different exercises for a while. Without knowing why you're doing these things, however, you would likely find your interest in the practice fizzling, and you would just try out a different program when next year's self-help books hit the shelves. The point of setting an intention for your practice is to assign a purpose to the work you're doing and to your life as a whole.

The purpose of this chapter is to teach you the significance of setting an intention for your practice, show you the different ways we can set intentions, and help you set an intention that will benefit your practice, your life, and society as a whole. Ron's passing played a significant role in how I set my intentions for my own life and how those intentions worked to benefit me and all those around me. Stories from several of my clients help to illustrate the difference between intentions that benefit us and those that don't.

what are the different kinds of intentions?

When observing people's choices as they relate to morality and ethics, it makes sense to define intentions as "good" or "bad." It may surprise you, though, to learn that when changing your life to find greater health and happiness, you need to consider more than just whether your intentions are good. You may have good intentions for practicing yoga, but your good intentions can still lack the necessary qualities you need to create change. If your intentions don't serve your ultimate purpose, then you might struggle to follow through with the practice over the length of time needed. To enjoy the benefits of the practice outlined in this book, you'll need to make sure your intentions are not just good but beneficial as well.

Below is an explanation of the different ways we can shape our intentions so that they are of genuine benefit to us.

MAKE YOUR INTENTIONS USEFUL

I had left the fashion industry to avoid having my career fade into obscurity through repeating the same jobs and getting gigs for older models. I had entered the restaurant and perfume businesses and was experiencing certain amounts of success and failure with those ventures—actually, more failures than successes. I had imagined that my contacts from the fashion industry would give me the platform for success and that I could ride my association with other famous people for my own benefit. That was naive. It turned out that Ron was right: I wasn't doing this work for any reason other than personal, selfish gain.

This is an example of an intention based on goals that served only my own needs. While my intention was not destructive in the sense of intending harm to others, neither was it useful. An intention that focuses only on our individual well-being entrenches us in the material world. It is detrimental to our path toward balance and happiness. If instead of owning a restaurant only because it seemed like the easiest way to make a lot of money, I had committed myself to that venture because I loved the act of facilitating the patrons' pleasure and nutrition through food, then I not only would have had useful intentions for pursuing my happiness, but I also would have created a better restaurant as well.

Useful intentions are made both to benefit one's own well-being and to affect others in a positive way. Since we depend on other people to sustain ourselves through shared experiences in business, socializing, and love, we must share the benefits of our growth. In business, a useful intention would be to start a vocation that benefits the environment and so is beneficial to all living beings. An intention that isn't useful would be to make as much money as possible no matter the effect on the planet or living things. In relationships, a useful intention would be to meet someone with the purpose of wanting to share mutually enjoyable moments together, and an intention that isn't useful would be to use that person for personal, physical, or mental gratification. Conducting business for easy money and physically gratifying ourselves may not be considered immoral, but these acts keep us entrenched in the dense material plane and impede our progress toward contentment and happiness. The state of the environment and the high divorce rate in our culture are a testament to the high number of intentions that aren't useful.

How can we have useful intentions as we practice discovering our inner guru? After Ron's passing, I came to the decision that I needed to listen to his wisdom and find my purpose through a spiritual practice. I had been going to ashrams and workshops for a number of years, but my participation in such things was sporadic, inconsistent, and not on a daily basis. I pursued spiritual growth only when it was convenient for me or when I was reading the latest spiritual book or encountering new teachings. Once I set the intention to find my practice after Ron's death, I wound up pursuing various tools on a regular basis regardless of whether I felt like doing them or not. I took an active role in practicing postures, breathing techniques, dietary behaviors, and modified sleeping habits. I committed to these practices for many years instead of just reading about them and applying them in the short term.

If you read this book from cover to cover and never experiment with a single exercise or try practicing a suggested routine, I consider it a failed teaching effort on my part and a waste of time on yours. The useful intention for a spiritual practice is to actually try it for some years so you can observe the impact it has on your life. In regard to this book, a useful intention is first of all to read and understand it but then also to try the practice out and see if it benefits you. If, after committing yourself to it for some time, you find that this practice doesn't serve you, then by all means find another practice to explore through a different book or resource. But remember, like the tallest and strongest trees that take hundreds of years to mature, you also are on a journey of exploration and spiritual growth and will require a lot of practice before becoming mature. Since you are reading this book, you have already demonstrated your willingness to grow and will therefore be likely to find success.

SPECIFY YOUR INTENTIONS

To be beneficial, intentions need to be specific rather than vague. While Ron's passing had inspired me to set useful intentions for my life, it was unclear for several years how those intentions would manifest themselves. After settling down in New York, I pursued yoga teacher training as well as reflexology training. They signified my new determination to find a healthy and spiritual practice, but I had signed up for them simply because I didn't know what else to do with myself. The information I learned was relevant and important, but because I had only a vague sense of why I was there, I did not learn all I could and was not able to apply the information in a beneficial way. I did have a certificate, but it represented less what I knew than what I had yet to learn.

A vague intention is a beneficial action that may not be related to our personal goals in any precise way. There is nothing wrong or harmful with having vague intentions, but there is nothing particularly helpful either. Vague intentions may cause distractions that end up costing us and others a lot of time, money, and energy. If I had been less vague in my intentions when I began my training on the yogic path, I might have found my true calling even earlier.

The opposite of a vague intention is, of course, a specific one. A specific intention not only reflects our goals in a precise way but also challenges us to understand what we really and truly want in accomplishing those goals. When I realized that I wasn't satisfied with the amount of information I had obtained from the various trainings I had done, I decided to research the different types of spiritual and medicinal paths that were available. In order to decide what I wanted to study, I had to repeatedly challenge myself to determine what I wanted, why I wanted it, how I was willing to get it, and how I was going to use it. If my vague intention was to pursue an Eastern, holistic path, then my specific intention was to immerse myself in a yoga and Ayurveda environment that eliminated distractions and could be taught to other people. If I had never gotten specific with my intentions, then today I might very well be floating around—but not levitating.

Since you have picked up this book and are trying the practices contained within it, the structure laid out here has helped you define your goal and think about how to pursue it. What this book can't tell you, however, is why you have this goal in the first place. Below we will explore how to set an intention that is useful and specific, and you will also have an opportunity to solidify why this work is important to you.

the three steps for setting an intention

The following process will show you how to set a useful and specific intention for pursuing your practice as defined by this book. It can also be applied while pursuing other goals as well. In fact, the more you practice the act of setting intentions, the more you'll understand the purpose of these goals.

STEP 1. ASK YOURSELF:
WHY IS CREATING CHANGE WORTH THE EFFORT?

In the previous section I suggested that one important component of this process is determining why you want to change in the first place. Determining why you want to practice is like building the foundation for a house; if you don't set the foundation well, the rest of the structure will eventually fall to the ground. Over the years clients have come to me with a variety of goals, and we have worked together to discover their intentions. Julie came to me to lose weight because she didn't feel her husband found her sexually desirable anymore. Dave wanted me to treat him for depression and diabetes; he wanted to make a change but was not sure how. Each of them had different intentions, and in order to work together, we needed to discover the reason why they had this goal of working on themselves.

Julie had the goal of losing weight because she wasn't feeling sexually satisfied in her marriage. She concluded that her husband would give her more attention and be attracted to her only if she looked a certain way. While there is nothing wrong with wanting to feel attractive, Julie was basing all of her frustrations on this one aspect of her life. Had our conversation ended there, Julie would have remained in the dark about her deeper reasons for wanting to create change. Through discussing it some more, Julie realized that she had been frustrated with the sexual aspects of her marriage well before she had put on any weight. With a little prompting, she determined that her real intentions were to feel healthy and good about herself as well as be warmer and more affectionate toward her husband.

Dave had more long-term goals than Julie, but they were not particularly specific. As we talked, it came to light that he worked at home and didn't really see his friends, family, or anyone else on a regular basis. He felt a certain amount of pain in his lower back and had difficulty breathing, to the point of disrupting his sleep. After discussing these issues, we revisited his reasons for coming to me, and he then decided that he wanted to change because he wanted to feel healthy and balanced so that he could feel better about the role he played in other people's lives.

Both of these people had reasons why they wanted to develop a practice, but if they had begun working without refining those reasons, it is likely they would not have continued on the path. In order to implement and sustain change, our reasons for our goals must be specific. Julie had specific intentions for practicing but was limited in her thinking about how it would be beneficial and whom it would benefit. Dave had useful intentions in wanting to feel better and be healed but wasn't specific enough in how he wanted to change and also hadn't thought about how his change could benefit his family and friends. I am pleased to report that after practicing with useful and specific intentions, Julie enjoyed the byproduct of losing some weight while she grew into a much more satisfying relationship with her husband, and Dave alleviated much of his pain and found new and exciting ways to relate to his friends and family.

STEP 2. CONTEMPLATE YOUR REASON

Contemplation often sounds foreign, doesn't it? Many of us have an image of contemplation that includes an ancient person in robes and sandals sitting atop a mountain in Tibet reflecting on all of humanity. You may be surprised to learn, however, that contemplation is probably one of the

why go out?

To teach yourself how to develop useful and specific intentions, use the following exercise the next time you plan to accept an invitation to attend a social gathering like a party or are asked to spend time with a particular friend or acquaintance. When someone invites you out, ask yourself why you're choosing to accept the invitation.

Some intentions for accepting this invitation may not be useful, such as wanting to avoid being alone on a Saturday night, having a good gossip session over drinks, or simply wanting to go out and make contacts for improving business. In contrast, useful intentions will not just satisfy your needs but also consider the needs of others, such as wanting to share an enjoyable experience with the other partygoers, being a source of comfort to someone who needs you, and looking to find people who share your philosophy of sound business practices.

This exercise is designed to help us understand our motives and why we form the habits we do. If we accept invitations and do other things just for our own benefit, it is unlikely that we will find genuine satisfaction from them. Behaviors that stem from a fear of being alone or avoiding some undesirable situation do not take into account other people's experiences. The more spiritually beneficial choice, in contrast, will consider the needs of others along with our own. If you find that your desire to accept an invitation is simply to satisfy your own selfish needs, then consider either not going or forming a different intention that includes those you will be interacting with. Selfish actions are fearful and are limited in results. Selfless actions are bountiful and result in true happiness for all.

easiest parts of this entire practice to understand. In its simplest terms, contemplation is just leaving aside a question for a certain period of time and letting the answer reveal itself on its own.

One of the reasons contemplation seems intimidating is that it requires us to let go both of the desire to instantly know the answer and also of our control over finding it without delay. We're so used to instantly finding other kinds of answers through Internet search engines like Google that we expect to find all our answers immediately. We're a culture that loves to intellectualize and analyze, and we're gratified when we figure things out. We go to tremendous lengths to hash things out, dissect them, and even beat them to death. All of these actions, however, are the opposite of contemplation, and we can drive ourselves crazy trying harder and harder to find answers that remain elusive. If we were truly to contemplate a question, we would just let it go until the answer is ready to come out.

Let's say you are trying to choose a preschool for your child to attend and have researched several places. You learn that you need to make a decision by a month before the first day of school to satisfy the various programs' admissions requirements. If in the time you have between researching schools and deciding on one you keep rereading brochures, asking friends about their children's experiences, and going through a dozen what-if scenarios that involve your child not getting a good education, then you're intellectualizing the question and not contemplating it.

To instead contemplate this question, first do your research, and then

dinner and contemplation

The next time you decide to go out with a friend or partner to a dinner and a movie, plan to go to the movie first. Before you arrive at the theater, talk with your friend to come up with three different restaurants that you would enjoy eating at afterward. Refrain from deciding on one of them. Take a moment, of course, to explain to your friend why you're doing this, and invite him or her to try the exercise as well. Then go and watch the movie and just enjoy the story without thinking about your upcoming dinner. Once the movie is over, see if one of the three restaurants has revealed itself as being a more desirable choice than the others. If a different answer has revealed itself to your friend, then you can try settling the disagreement through fisticuffs. Just kidding.

This exercise includes watching a movie and, as you might have surmised, doesn't seem like a particularly awakened thing to do. The point of the movie is to create an environment that allows you *not* to think about restaurants because you're focusing on the movie instead. Generally, your contemplations will not include relying on distractions like movies and other entertainments, but for this first step you can give yourself permission to zone out for a bit. You can then use this practice to find a school for your child, decide whether or not to go on a date, determine how much money to lend to someone, pick a new job, or make any other type of decision, no matter how seemingly big or small. The first, very important step in your contemplation is not to stress yourself out trying to come up with the right answer.

stop thinking about the different schools at all. You might need to put the question down for a few days or a month before the right feeling guides you to the best decision. However long it takes, the decision will happen at the right time. You will likely find exactly the right school for your child, and it will result from not trying so hard. Contemplation includes relaxing the mind and allowing a higher feeling to take over. When this happens, your spontaneity and energy will emerge, and things will turn out even better than they would have if the intellectual mind had been in charge.

Once you have asked yourself why you want to take up a spiritual practice, it will serve you to contemplate your answer before moving forward. There is no set amount of time for how long this contemplation should last, but if you're eager to begin then I recommend you take at least a few days to not think about it before moving on to the next step. On page 38 there is a simple exercise to help you understand the nature of contemplation.

STEP 3. ASK YOURSELF:
ARE YOU BEING TRUE TO THE ANSWERS YOU'VE FOUND?

Once you've asked yourself why you're doing something and contemplated your possible answers, it is then time to observe whether or not you're being true to the answers you've found. Like the act of contemplation, this act of observing truth may seem intimidating, but it's really nothing more than asking yourself if you really do feel as true what you declared to be your reason for doing the activity. If you decided to begin this practice because you wanted to be healthier and improve your relationship with your spouse, then once you've begun your practice you need to consider whether or not you are being honest about your intentions. For example, let's say that through this practice you attained greater physical health and have experienced a surge of energy. If, instead of simply enjoying your new vitality, you tell someone to change their life in a similar way, then your actions are not honestly reflecting useful intentions.

This step is more open-ended than the previous two, as you will be observing yourself not just within a fixed period of time but instead over the course of your practice. Given the longer time frame, consider setting a reminder for yourself to take a few minutes every couple of weeks or every month to reflect on your original intentions.

You might notice that I do not offer a method for deciding whether or not you are being true to your intentions. This is because you are the only one who can know, and there's no yes-or-no answer. It is your responsibility to observe the significance of your thoughts and actions. In the next part of the book we'll delve further into the act of observation and how it can be used to more fully realize our balance and happiness.

Setting an intention for yourself not only lays the groundwork for your practice, but it also helps you investigate the truth behind your actions and whether or not you're serving yourself in whatever decisions you make. At the beginning, certain decisions may seem more difficult, and others will be so easy to make that you'll wonder why you never found those answers before. You'll begin to notice that when you set the proper intentions for yourself, everything will become an expression of your practice. You will do things because they help you and others to feel good, and you will continue to grow with each day you're alive. Your practice, in turn, will become an expression of who you are.

. . .

Several years after I finished my first training in India, I was in Paris working with a client at an office building in the 2nd arrondissement. After we were done for the day, I found myself wandering north, though without any real idea of where I was going. After about an hour, I found myself in a familiar location.

I began walking along a canal and turned off into a side street. I stopped and looked through a window that I had looked through many times before. I saw an old woman serving customers and a display case at the counter filled with all sorts of organic treats. There was a display of postcards, and a man in a green jumpsuit and a baseball hat was looking at it. The man turned to look out the window at me and smiled.

Ron always did enjoy looking at all those postcards from so many different places, I thought, for it was a reminder of the contentment he had finally found by living out the rest of his life in Paris. I closed my eyes and reopened them to see a storefront that was closed for the day and must have replaced the café years ago. As I had made it my practice to live for the present moment and to value my relationships with those still with me, I hadn't thought of Ron for quite a long time. Though it may have

set your intention for your practice

As I said earlier, setting your intention for your practice is similar to laying the foundation for building a house: without the necessary groundwork, the structure is at risk of falling apart. Because of this, it is important that you set your intention right now before moving forward with reading the rest of the book and trying additional exercises. I have provided a suggested outline for how to set an intention for your practice below.

1. **Ask yourself why you have a goal.** State to yourself why you want to use the tools in this book to practice, starting with the words, "I am going to practice because . . ." If it helps you, you may write this statement down. Ask yourself if the reason you have stated will have a long-term impact, will affect others in a positive way, and is specific. If it doesn't satisfy all of these things, consider revising the statement.

2. **Contemplate your reason.** Once you have refined your reason to make sure it is useful and specific, let go of the statement and contemplate it for at least several days. If you feel comfortable with not thinking about it for a week, give that a try. Be sure to make an appointment with yourself to revisit your statement so that you don't risk the chance of losing interest in this exercise. If you do forget about it, this is a sign that the task at hand may not be as important to you at the moment as you had thought.

3. **Observe the truth of your intention.** When you have practiced contemplation, revisit the statement and take a moment—but just a moment—to explore whether or not it's true. Revisit this statement every couple of weeks or every month as you continue on with the remainder of the exercises outlined in this book. Real practice is not bound to the limits of time, though, so be liberal and generous with how much time you give yourself.

been a bit of a departure from how I preferred to live, this moment of nostalgia served as a reminder of what set me on this path in the first place.

It was my intention to share and live in joy.

fill in the blank

As you move along into Part Two, you will begin to build a practice from the ground up. Without first setting a useful intention to practice, though, it is likely for this reading experience to be little more than entertainment. Before moving on to Part Two, take the time to set an intention for your practice as per the exercise on page 41.

foundation

the practice of nonviolence

3

kindness toward ourselves and others

WHEN I SAW MY FATHER coming out of the house, I thought I was in trouble. He didn't want me playing soccer in the street, for he thought it was dangerous for eight-year-olds to be playing in the line of fast-moving traffic. As a boy in 1975 Iran, however, I was interested in little else but soccer.

It turned out, though, that my father wasn't coming out to punish me. Though he did send a glare my way, he got into his car and began pulling out of the driveway, perhaps running some errands before heading off to work. As he was backing out, the boys from the soccer game began to quickly clear the street because a man on a motorcycle was speeding toward us. I was following them over toward the stream that flowed beside my house when I heard the loud crunching sound behind me. I knew what had happened before I even turned around. Sure enough, the man on the motorcycle had collided with my father, speeding into the car's rear fender. The fender was smashed in and the motorcycle was totaled, but the man's look of despair was the ugliest result of the whole accident.

After he inspected the damage, my father invited the man into our house. For once, I was happy to choose the house over playing soccer in the street for it gave me a front-row seat to watch what would happen next. I followed them in.

After my mother served tea, my dad found out that the man had been on his way to find work in the city and not only didn't have any money to pay my dad back for the damage but couldn't even afford to fix or replace his motorcycle. The man looked miserable when he said this, and he didn't even touch his tea.

My father watched this display, inspecting the man from over the brim of his cup and saucer. He took a thoughtful sip, and I waited for him to pronounce the sentence.

"Don't worry about the car," my father said. My mother, standing at the kitchen counter, said nothing, though she did take a bit more interest in the conversation after this.

The man's eyes darted up to meet my father's, unsure if he had heard correctly. He remained quiet, perhaps fearful of disturbing his sudden shift of fortune, though his posture straightened a bit.

"How much did you pay for the bike?" my father asked.

"Thirty thousand rials," the man said, the equivalent of four hundred dollars. He must have suddenly remembered how much money this was for his shoulders began to sag again.

"Okay," my father said, "I will give you the money." He left to go to his bedroom, where I imagined he was getting the cash. I looked at my mother, thinking that I must have misheard. Her face looked nonplussed, which told me nothing.

My father returned from the bedroom with a handful of cash and gave it to the man, who hadn't stirred since hearing my father would give him the money. He held the money in his hand and stared at it a moment, and then said something inaudible.

"Excuse me?" my father asked.

"Th-thank you," said the man. They worked out getting the motorcycle picked up and getting the man a ride into the city, and after the man thanked my parents a few hundred more times, he left and everything settled down again. My father still had to get to work, and since my mother simply said that my father would explain, I had to wait until the next day to ask him about what had happened.

"Why did you give him the money, Daddy?"

"Because, Cameron, he needed it."

Iran in 1975 was not like America today—or like my mother's native England, for that matter. People didn't use auto insurance, they didn't sue each other, and they settled things without the use of the authorities or other third parties. Often, someone in this man's situation would be expected to be in debt to someone more influential like my father for however long the more influential person deemed it necessary. The fact that my father chose to settle the situation in the man's favor, however, had less to do with his being Iranian and more to do with the fact that he saw it as an opportunity to practice kindness toward another.

When my father explained this to me, I said I understood.

"Cameron."

"Yes, Daddy?"

"There's one other thing I must tell you."

I waited, wondering what other sage advice he might share.

"No more playing football in the street."

"Oh." I paused. "Yes, Daddy."

. . .

Years later, in 2007, I was in India shooting a documentary. I had already been to this country several times in pursuit of my training and had decided to develop a film based on my studies. The film documented the journey of two Americans overwhelmed with disease and personal strife and showed how Ayurveda and the principles of natural medicine could help them in a way that Western medicine could not. We were to be in India shooting material for about a month and a half, and I was there with a crew of ten people.

After about two weeks, my girlfriend joined us for a few days. On her second day we visited a medicine man who lived a number of miles from a small town in a remote area atop a mountain. After we had interviewed him and gathered some shots on film, we went down the mountain and found a tiny wooden tea hut.

The tea hut could perhaps fit two or three people inside it if those people didn't expect to move their arms or legs. A few chairs and tables were set up outside the hut, and otherwise the patrons had to sit on nearby rocks.

As my girlfriend and I were moving toward two of the chairs near this little hut, one of the other patrons walked toward the stand, perhaps for a refill. He was a quick little man with sure, confident steps. He was far smaller than most of the members of my crew. My girlfriend and I moved to get out of his path, but he stopped in front of us and with all his might smacked my girlfriend across the face. He then looked around at our group, all of whose eyes were now on him.

The events that followed happened rather quickly.

One crew member went for the man and grabbed his shirt. Two more lunged for the man, and between the three of them they tackled him to the ground. One of them proceeded to punch him in the face. Other members of my crew watched as two of them began to kick the man in the torso and legs. I looked at my girlfriend, who seemed to be in shock, but other than the red mark on her cheek where the man had slapped her, she looked okay. I went for the large group, pushed my way through to the man on the ground, and placed my body between the man and everyone else until the fighting had stopped.

"Enough," I said.

"But he just went up to her and slapped her without provocation!" one of them protested.

"Still, though, he should not be beaten like this." I remained between them and the man.

"You and she are our guests here," he continued. "That is not how we treat our guests in India."

"Perhaps," I said, "but he should be taken to the police for them to handle it."

Nitin, our cinematographer, stepped in and took the man to the side.

The others remained unconvinced, but they didn't stand in the way as the man was brought to a car to sit until we figured out how to notify the authorities. Given how far we were from any towns or cities, we were going to have to wait a while for someone to arrive.

violence

We live in a violent culture. Violence, as it relates to the intentions of this book, is a harmful action directed against oneself or another, either physically or mentally. We experience violence in response to negative emotions, and these emotional reactions lead to pain and hinder our spiritual growth. Many of us associate violence with overt physical actions that inflict physical harm on another, such as shooting or stabbing someone. While inflicting physical harm is very much a part of violence, it is only one type. We commit an act of violence toward another whenever we yell at someone, wish harm on them, or even gossip about a person's flaws behind his or her back. We inflict violence upon ourselves not only when we cause harm to our own bodies, such as when we smoke or overeat, but also when we berate ourselves for a mistake or tell ourselves that no one will ever love us.

Given this definition and these examples, it's obvious that there is an abundance of violence in our culture. Whether in the form of harm inflicted on ourselves or another, the frequency of acts of violence is eroding our potential for living a life of awareness, peace, and joy. In this chapter we will examine the difference between physical violence, which is the physical harm of oneself or another, and mental violence, which is thinking or believing something harmful in relation to oneself or another. Violence affects us all, but there are things we can do to overcome this as an obstacle in our relationships with ourselves and everyone around us. One question I encourage my clients to ask is: How are such acts detrimental to our well-being?

The two stories I told at the beginning of this chapter demonstrate how my own relationship with violence has evolved over the years. The story of the man who crashed his motorcycle recalled the first time I encountered a situation with the potential for significant conflict. My father, however, not only did not pursue the conflict but regarded the situation as an opportunity to help another human being. In contrast, today's Western culture might deem it necessary to mete out justice, making the man pay for damage or fining him for reckless driving.

My father's actions that day had a significant influence on how I handled conflicts once I reached adulthood. I got into my own share of conflicts as I got older and did not follow my father's example, yet by setting the proper intentions and discovering my practice, I responded to the man slapping my girlfriend in an entirely different way. When some of my crew began to beat the man, they were coming to my girlfriend's defense, but they were still perpetuating the conflict through their actions. My decision to put an end to the conflict grew out of a practice of nonviolence. Though it took a number of years to integrate such a practice into my everyday thoughts and actions, the practice of nonviolence emulates the very intentions my father put forth thirty years prior. The second story shows aggressive physical violence, but the work you will do in this chapter will be centered on more nuanced forms of violence toward yourself and others.

how violence affects us all

Violence, as I said, is harm done either physically or mentally. We can hit someone in the face (a physical act of violence), or we can think that we want to hit that person in the face (a mental act of violence).

Both physical and mental violence provoke reactions. My film crew felt righteous anger when they saw the man in India slapping a woman, and they reacted by ganging up on the man. Because they reacted with the emotion of anger, they too acted with violence.

When an act of violence is committed, those of us who don't set the intention to practice awareness inevitably react with some sort of negative emotion: anger, fear, worry, sadness, grief, despair, and so forth. When we experience one of these emotions, we experience a form of pain or suffering.

Pain is our body's way of sending a message to the brain that we must conduct a new and different action for healing. The sensation of pain, like all other sensations we experience, is relayed to the brain by our nervous system and the many millions of cells known as neurons. When we experience one of the negative emotions, be it fear of a physical injury we just sustained or anger toward someone we feel has wronged us, our neurons deliver the message to the brain that something is wrong. Given how much of the nervous system's activity is conducted within the brain and spinal cord, it makes sense that experiencing some form of violence inflicted by ourselves or another can lead to problems in related parts of our anatomy, such as our head, neck, and back. In yogic terms, pain represents an energy blockage somewhere in our system.

physical violence

As noted earlier, for the sake of exploring how to practice a life free of violence, we will focus on the more subtle forms of physical violence that we may engage in day to day. If you are inclined to strike others in random attacks of aggression, as did the man in India, then by all means consider the steps of the practice outlined in this book, but also consider enlisting the help of others to overcome this behavior.

In the practice outlined in this book, we are more concerned with a physical act that creates disharmony in the body and mind and can therefore lead to pain and suffering. Physical practices like smoking, overeating, and drinking alcohol, sodas, or coffee tax the body's ability to function. Regularly eating junk food, fast food, and processed foods taxes the digestive system and drains us of our vitality. Having cosmetic surgery done on our bodies requires the body to endure severe trauma and creates an abundance of pain. Putting ourselves in places filled with intense stimuli, such as an overwhelming work environment, a loud bar, or a shooting range, can create an abundance of stress and induce the body's fight-or-flight instincts unnecessarily. Bodybuilding and other extreme conditioning exercises put stress on our muscles and joints to the point of causing potential injury and a blockage of energy. Even participating in unsportsmanlike competition in athletics, shouting at the visiting team as a spectator of an event, or killing animals for sport can subject the body to stress and send a message to the brain that the body must compensate for physical, mental, and emotional disharmony. When we have endured a series of violent physical acts perpetrated either by ourselves or another, we run the risk of experiencing severe problems with our health and well-being.

Helen, one of my clients, is an example of a person who experienced pain as the result of physical violence. Both of Helen's parents had a genetic predisposition toward obesity and passed these genes on to her. When Helen was a young girl, her father made her chase her mother around the block so that the physical activity would help her and her mother lose weight. As a result of this and other forms of treatment, Helen began to hide the unhealthy foods she liked to eat from her father, began hiding from her father outright, and even thought of committing suicide when she was eight years old. She continued to develop an unhealthy relationship with food as she grew up, and as a grown woman she disliked her body, disliked herself, and continued to suffer from morbid obesity. The doctors she saw diagnosed her with attention deficit disorder, arthritis, candida, and migraines. She experienced severe cramping during her period and got violent sinus headaches when she experienced negative thoughts—which she did on a regular basis.

Helen was not physically abused by her father in the form of beatings or sexual assault, but she did form an unhealthy relationship with her body in part through the extreme measures her father enforced to make her thin. Instead of being healthy, she was put through the physical actions of required exercise, which resulted in the emotional reactions of guilt, despair, and helplessness. She became convinced she wasn't good enough as is, and at the best of times she physically abused herself through an improper diet of junk food and at worst almost tried to take her own life. These numerous acts of physical violence led her to think she was unwanted as a human being. If Helen was ever to experience happiness, it was necessary for her to implement changes in her life. Later in this chapter, we will see how she made this happen.

mental violence

Earlier I described mental violence as thinking or believing something harmful in relation to oneself or another. Even if we never intend to commit an act of physical harm, we might think how much we would like to do so, and this act can have a negative effect. We might say to ourselves, "I'd really like to punch him in the face," when someone makes an offensive comment or, "What are you looking at?" when we feel that someone is staring at us inappropriately. We can watch a movie that uses humor to attack another person, and when we revel not just in the expression of humor but in how this humor has succeeded in embarrassing the person being made fun of, we're joining in the attack. We commit mental violence when we gossip and judge people for not living up to our expectations. These and many other thoughts we have against another person are acts of mental violence.

It may not be difficult to understand how wishing someone harm, even if we do not act upon that wish, constitutes an act of mental violence. However, let's consider more nuanced situations. Let's say that you're running a bit late for an important lunch meeting and are stressing about the time. You berate yourself for not being diligent enough with your schedule and decide that you might have to fire your assistant for not getting you out the door quickly enough. After cursing to yourself about a group of tourists who felt they had to walk in front of you four abreast as they slowly snapped pictures of everything they saw for three blocks, you finally make it to the restaurant. You arrive at the front of the establishment at the same moment as a man dressed impeccably in a custom-tailored suit bought with the salary of a job that you could never get, and when you sacrifice three whole seconds of time to let him through the door first, he doesn't even thank you for your politeness. You shake your head behind his back and think the phrase, "Um, you're welcome?" as you finally make it to the host with his reservation booklet. There you find that your lunch date is running late. You roll your eyes as you decide that you can't rely on anyone to be on time anymore. As you sit at the table, you massage your temples, feeling a headache beginning to form. You order a stiff drink to remove yourself from the ordeal.

Has something like this ever happened to you?

Many times, when we're under stress or feeling negative emotions, we may fill our heads with all sorts of mental violence. In the hypothetical situation above, you committed acts of mental violence when you berated yourself for being late, blamed your assistant, cursed the tourists, envied the affluent man in the suit, resented the man for not thanking you, became impatient with your lunch date for not being on time, and finally polluted your body and mind with alcohol. While this example may be exaggerated, it still shows how prominent mental violence is in our busy, high-stressed lives.

You might also note that this example ended with you experiencing a headache. Much as a physically violent act, such as abusing one's body with excessive eating, can progress into thoughts based in pain or anxiety ("I don't like my body and I'll always be fat"), mentally violent acts such as resenting the person who didn't say thank you when you held open the door can turn into a physical form of pain such as a headache—or, over many years of headaches, develop into a more severe illness such as a tumor.

Rebecca used to be physically active and healthy. However, she went through an awful divorce that included a contentious custody battle over her daughter and the challenge of reestablishing her financial independence from scratch. Along with resenting her ex-husband and wishing for her daughter to dislike her father as much as Rebecca did, she also began to feel contempt for everything her life stood for. She began to obsess over all of the things that were wrong with her life and felt jealous of friends and family members who had been more successful in creating a healthy and happy home life. She grew fearful of what could happen next, and in her head a simple mantra ran day in and day out: "I don't like myself or my life."

Though this may have been a genetic inevitability, it also seems significant that within a few years of getting divorced, Rebecca began developing, as diagnosed by her doctor, early symptoms of multiple sclerosis.

Given that multiple sclerosis (MS) is a condition of the nervous system, it makes sense that her body would in part respond to all of her negative thoughts in this way. When one commits acts of mental violence, the nervous system alerts the body that the mind is imbalanced. The more energy the body spends on healing that imbalance, the weaker it becomes. This internal fight further taxes the body, thus setting the stage for illness. A disease like MS, while an extreme case, is an example of what may happen. Along with MS, Rebecca was diagnosed with hyperthyroidism and required medication to treat it, suffered from hemorrhoids, suffered from an increase in weight, experienced heavy bleeding during her period, suffered from back pain, and was so constipated that she moved her bowels only every two to four days.

While Helen experienced acts of physical violence in the form of enforced activity and in turn suffered from negative thoughts, Rebecca committed many acts of mental violence in the form of bitterness and self-pity and in turn suffered from a debilitating disease. In both cases, though, the women's bodies went to war against themselves because they were depleted from constantly having to spend energy to heal instead of being able to maintain the proper homeostasis. Each woman experienced significant pain and suffering as a result of these imbalances. In the next section, we'll learn about the practice of nonviolence—how we can use this practice for better living, and how such a practice helped both Helen and Rebecca to implement real change.

nonviolence

The scriptures of yoga, which date back many centuries, identify nonviolence as a practice that centers on the avoidance of killing or injuring other living beings. The scriptures suggest that if we cause harm to one living thing, we are actually causing harm to ourselves. This practice may manifest in contemporary day-to-day life in many ways, but it is refraining from injuring ourselves and others that informs much of the practice taught in this chapter.

The intention to abstain from acts of physical and mental violence is based on the assumption that every living being is a part of the natural order of all things on earth. This truth of a collective can be called many things, be it nature, the Spirit, or for those with religious backgrounds, God.

Consider, then, the vilest example of a human being, such as Hitler, Stalin, or Pol Pot. Most of us probably think of these men as evil, detestable people deserving every negative association made with their names. By contrast, teachings derived from Eastern systems such as yoga and Buddhism consider all people to be enlightened beings who have the responsibility to awaken themselves to that enlightenment through useful, good intentions and practice. Observing a practice of nonviolence allows one to regard even these apparently evil men as having this potential but having strayed so far from this practice that they destroyed other lives rather than celebrated them.

Any form of violence creates pain, and it is our job to practice eliminating as much pain as possible while in this material form. By practicing this lifestyle, we can create greater love, peace, and joy during our time on earth. But trying to end conflicts through more violence means we have not grasped that all people belong to the same humanity. For instance, while my crew might have wanted to end the conflict that began when my girlfriend was attacked, their decision to resolve it with another act of violence required them to consider the man who slapped her as not being a part of humanity but at a lower level of being. The man was certainly doing inappropriate things, but from a nonviolent perspective he was acting out of ignorance. It's possible that by preventing him from being beaten by my crew, I helped him to grow away from the ignorance that triggered his volatile behavior. My dad had the option to take advantage of his influence and place demands on the man who crashed his motorcycle in order to further his own gain, but he opted to help the man instead and possibly fostered a greater sense of goodwill.

The question, then, is how do we begin to practice nonviolence? It probably seems like a tall order to consider the man in India—let alone Hitler—as deserving of anything but violence as retribution for what he did. It is important to remember, though, that a nonviolent practice does not begin with deciding that the man who killed six million people might not have been such a bad guy after all. Instead, it begins with observing our own sense of violence toward ourselves and others and developing a greater love of our own bodies, minds, and place on earth. Through this practice, we can then develop a similar awareness of the actions of others.

I had the opportunity to work with Helen, whose father had forced her to engage in exercise to lose weight, for a month and a half. As her obstacles were based on a negative perception of herself, I took her through a regimen that would nurture her and help her to end the war she was waging on her body through poor diet choices and a sedentary lifestyle. I began with an Ayurvedically inspired routine that included herbal therapies, specific yoga postures that would help nurture her body and balance anger-related energy, and breathing exercises to help her build her metabolism. Perhaps most important of all, I had her completely simplify her

physical nonviolence toward yourself

You already know that behaviors like eating too much and consuming intoxicating substances are detrimental to your well-being. However, as much as we all know that certain behaviors aren't good for us, we still engage in them all the same. We might know that smoking is bad for us, but our addiction makes it nearly impossible to quit. We might know that it's best not to gorge ourselves on Thanksgiving, but we do it anyway. We may get completely over-the-top competitive in playing a sport, even if it's just the friendly neighborhood league organized by friends in the community.

Knowing that it's going to happen again, I would like you to try something the next time you chain-smoke your way through an evening, eat three times as much food as what you need to satisfy your hunger, scream yourself hoarse at the opposing team, or any other physically violent behavior. Simply observe how you feel the following day. Do you have a midafternoon slump? Are you sore, tired, or lethargic? Are you hyperactive?

Is your mind thinking even more? Do you have difficulty sleeping? Make a mental note of how you feel.

A couple of days later, consider how you felt once again, and if you feel better now that you've put some time between your indulgence and the present moment. If you really do feel better, consider whether it will be worth it to regress into bad feelings the next time you're presented with an opportunity to burden your body with physical violence.

Please note that in presenting this exercise to you, I am in no way condoning a relapse into physically violent behaviors. In moving forward with your practice of nonviolence toward yourself, experiment with eliminating foods that may be bad for you, try sleeping at the same earlier time each night, and continue to notice any changes that occur in how you feel as you make more positive changes to your habits. Later in this book I will provide specific exercises related to food and physical activity that will provide you with the tools for making more positive choices in your lifestyle.

diet to eat only one full-sized meal a day at lunchtime. She supplemented this meal with juices at other times of the day, and the food she did eat was cooked thoroughly to aid digestion. At the end of the month and a half, she had no candida, no migraines, no arthritis, no stomach issues, no menstrual pains, and she of course reduced her weight. Her body was happy because she was treating it well.

Rebecca, the woman who was developing symptoms of MS, was a client whom I saw over the course of twenty-one days. To help her resolve the challenges she had encountered with her disease and other conditions, I had her modify her lifestyle in a variety of ways. I treated her with herbal medicines, yoga postures to build confidence, and breathing exercises to

mental nonviolence toward yourself

Rebecca's mental violence toward herself culminated in repeatedly stating that she didn't like herself. This exercise is a particularly simple one, in that your only assignment is to notice acts of mental violence that you commit against yourself in the form of negative, self-defeating thoughts. Practicing nonviolence in response to such thoughts is similar to reprogramming a machine to perform a different function. However, because we send so many messages to our brains in any given day, this type of reprogramming takes a lot of practice.

The first step is to mentally prepare a list of negative thoughts that you say to yourself in any given day. I do not advocate writing your lists down, as putting energy into that type of activity can be contrary to the work you're doing. Even if you think of only one or two negative thoughts, that is plenty to start with. Some examples of the kind of thoughts you might have include:

I'm out of shape.

I'll never amount to anything.

I'll always be alone.

I'll always be fat.

I'm not smart enough.

I don't have enough money.

I don't like the way I look.

I don't like the way I feel.

I'm always going to be tired.

I won't ever find success.

People don't understand me.

I don't have enough friends.

No one will ever love me.

I need something to make me happy.

As this exercise is a practice of abstention, the next step is for you to focus on removing this type of language from your inner monologue. This will happen over a long period of time, so your task is to observe the next time you say something to yourself that fits into the above list and to follow that thought with, "There's a better way."

You may notice that the response to the negative thought is not to use flowery language on yourself, make ambitious proclamations of positive affirmations, or use the threat of change. The entire concept of this practice is that there is a better way to live, and this exercise simply reiterates that in a literal way.

For example, let's say your mother is visiting you from out of town. While you have a great relationship, you see her as liking to nitpick about details of your life that, as a grown adult, you feel have no place in your conversations. This is especially the case when she visits, for she always makes a comment about whether or not there's enough food in the refrigerator or whether or not you've properly organized your closets. Rather than getting into an argument with her and saying

to yourself, "My mother won't ever understand me," use these types of comments as an opportunity to practice the exercise. When she says, "No wonder you can't find anything; look at the mess in your closet!" you can simply say to yourself, "This is what Yogi Cameron was talking about, so now I can change my thoughts." Then, because you're not dwelling on negative thoughts or how to answer back, you relieve yourself of useless, unproductive tension and place the focus back on your mother. You can now simply watch and allow her to be herself without the need to change her or tell her she is wrong. This begins the act of acceptance. Strangely enough, what often happens is that when you welcome such a comment because it gives you an opportunity to practice, it might not ever come.

Give this exercise a try the next time you think something negative about yourself. Keep in mind that each of us is likely to inflict pain on others when we are in pain ourselves.

foster calm in the nervous system. To relieve her constipation, I had her take one tablespoon of castor oil with warm water at night every two to three days for about two weeks. She was used to eating a lot of meat, and since meat takes a long time to digest and has little water content, I had her refrain from eating it. I encouraged her to cut out frozen and processed foods in favor of fresh fruits and vegetables and to eat two meals, at 11:00 a.m. and 5:00 p.m., instead of ending her three meals a day with dinner at 8:00 or 9:00 at night. I also suggested she go to sleep earlier, at around 10:00 p.m. At the end of the three weeks, her doctor stated that she no longer had a thyroid problem, her clothes started to feel big on her, she was going to the bathroom every day, and, most significantly, her overall energy was lighter and healthier than it had been when I first met her. She was well on her way to freeing herself of the violent thoughts that had plagued her since her divorce, and months later her doctor informed her that there were no more signs of MS.

nonviolence toward others

When we set the intention to practice nonviolence toward others, what we are really doing is committing ourselves to playing the part of objective witness to a conflict instead of reacting with our emotions. The first step of this practice is to present yourself with a situation that makes you upset or angry but that allows you to retain complete control over how and when you are exposed to it. This can happen when you turn on the television.

Think of a person on TV that you don't like. This may be a social commentator who uses the show's platform to promote a political agenda, a news reporter who you think wouldn't know a thing about the world if it wasn't presented to him or her on a teleprompter, or a cast member of a reality show who really annoys you by constantly yelling at the other cast members. Your task in considering this person is, simply put, to observe him or her.

Set an egg timer, stopwatch, or the alarm on your cell phone to go off three minutes after you have begun watching the problem personality. Watch the show as you normally would, allowing whatever emotions to come up that usually do. If what you're watching usually upsets you, then you might think, "I hate how that commentator always yells at his guests," or, "I can't stand how that news reporter dresses like a game show hostess instead of a journalist." When the three minutes are up, note to yourself three things that are on the screen, omitting all opinions and commentary. For example, instead of hating what is happening onscreen, you might think simply, "The commentator is yelling at his guest," or, "The news reporter is wearing red." When you simply state to yourself what you're seeing instead of adding commentary or expressing your distaste for it, you're practicing nonviolence.

Note how long it takes for you to revert back to feeling upset or opinionated in response to what you are seeing. Set the timer again for another three minutes, and when it goes off detach and observe once again. Continue this cycle for the remainder of the show.

When you've become more adept at sustaining your detachment from what you are seeing on the screen, feel free to experiment. Set the timer for ten minutes instead of three, and see if it's harder to detach when you're more invested in what is happening on the show. See if you can watch a whole TV show by doing nothing but observing what is on the screen.

While these examples demonstrate the benefits of practicing nonviolence, they also show how much work it can take to create this type of change in one's life. The good news, however, is that this type of practice can begin with very small steps and can be done on your own in a safe and nonthreatening way. In the next section I will share three exercises that will help you begin your own practice of nonviolence toward yourself and others.

When you move forward with your practice of nonviolence, it will be your job to observe your reactions to situations that would otherwise inspire you to project a form of violence toward that situation. Is there a co-worker or in-law whom you don't like? Use the tool of observation the next time this person does something to upset you. Do you have repeatedly negative thoughts about yourself that cause anxiety, stress, and depression? Remind yourself that there's another way to live, and instead of putting your attention on the easy way of remaining in your suffering, place it on the practice of change. Is there a physical activity that induces a sense of pain in you? Try modifying that activity until you no longer feel pain. You will be on your way to practicing nonviolence toward all living things.

. . .

Everything outside the tea hut had settled down a few minutes after the man had smacked my girlfriend. Although her head was still ringing, she seemed to have gotten past the shock of being attacked. I turned to her and said, "I would like you to consider talking to that man before he leaves."

"Why?" she asked. She looked very uncomfortable with this idea.

"I think it's important that you connect with him before he's turned over to the police. It may be an opportunity to learn why he did it in the first place."

She didn't look convinced that this was worth the awkwardness of facing this man again, but she was also used to me and my crazy yogic ideas and was always open to the idea that this was the right thing to practice. She nodded to me.

"You're coming with me," she said. I nodded back. Of course I was.

The man was sitting in the backseat of the car. His shirt was torn, and a trickle of blood had dried on his temple, but the most interesting thing was that his eyes were red from what must have been many tears. When he looked up at my girlfriend, he looked terrified.

"Sorry." he said. "Sorry, sorry, sorry." He began rocking in his seat.

My girlfriend continued to look at him, as though seeing his misery gave her more curiosity than apprehension.

"Why did you do that?" she asked him.

"No, no, sorry, sorry, sorry." He continued to rock back and forth.

"Why?" she asked again.

"Sorry." He didn't seem to know any other words.

She looked at me, her face impassive. She wasn't going to find out why this man did what he did, but rather than attack him or retaliate, she simply observed his reaction. Later on she would tell me that while she was still afraid when she went over to the car, seeing him in his awful state taught her that reacting to him in anger wasn't going to make the situation any better.

It was her practice of nonviolence.

fill in the blank

Non-violence is the first of Part Two's three basic practices, as it plays such a dominating role in our moment-to-moment lives. Try each of the three exercises provided in this chapter before moving on to chapter 4.

4 the practice of detachment

allowing what nature intends for us

HE PHOTOGRAPHER WAS TAKING a long time to review
our portfolios. Every once in a while he looked back up at my friend
Bruce and me. We had dropped in to his studio one afternoon in
1988 to show him our work. It was early in our modeling careers,
and we were hungry for bigger jobs. We were both wearing the same basic
"Buffalo Boys" look made popular by the stylist Ray Petri at the time:
Levi's 501 jeans, tight white T-shirt, a double-breasted leather jacket, and
shin-high biker boots.

"Indeed . . . *Sa se très cool* . . ." he said in his French accent as he flipped
through the pages.

At one point he closed my book and shoved it back in my arms without
looking at me. I raised my eyebrows to Bruce, who looked like he too was
wondering if we had done something to offend him. The photographer
had been doing a shoot for a magazine editorial, but it hadn't seemed like
we were interrupting his work. Besides, our agency had told us to come by
and show him our books that afternoon.

The photographer walked across the studio and spoke to a woman
standing there. He pointed at us and then brought her over to where we
were standing.

"This is what we need. I want these two guys."

"Wait—what?" the woman said. She looked nonplussed.

"The other boys aren't working for this shoot," he continued. "The women are formal, but having the men also wearing formalwear is too bland and obvious. I want contrast, I want these guys just the way they are, natural."

The woman, who by now I had surmised was the magazine's editor, looked at us with our darker features as well as our jeans and leather jackets.

"You're right," she said after a beat. "Make it happen."

Bruce and I got the job. The photographer felt that the blond, suit-wearing male models had too much in common with the women's more elegant haute couture look. The editorial was being shot to feature the made-to-order formality of these women, and so we, by dressing differently, would add more tension to the shoot and therefore draw more favorable attention to the women. We were so hungry for interesting work that given half a chance, and if the dresses hadn't been a size 1, we would have dressed in the ladies' wear and taken the place of the female models too. I was not being nasty, I just wanted work that was artistically challenging. The women were doing all of the interesting work in the business, and I wanted to receive as much attention as they did.

Things had begun picking up for my modeling career. I had begun working in the fashion industry in late 1986, and by 1988 I had worked a number of shows for French designers and had shot a few magazine editorials. My relatively dark features usually kept me away from the more commercial catalog shoots, and my agent in Paris almost never bothered to send me out for such gigs. With lips like mine, the only way for me to fit into those more commercial times would have been to model for Michelin—using my lips as tires!

This suited me fine. I had little interest in working in such a creative industry as a standard drone, and I wanted something larger and better than what had been accomplished by any male model up to that point. I wanted to ride the wave of growing supermodel fame that women like Claudia Schiffer and Christy Turlington had already begun to find. Magazine editorials were fine, but they weren't going to get me to the top of my profession. What I needed was an ad campaign with a big American designer.

"A major American designer wants to see you," my New York agent told me over the phone several weeks after Bruce and I had done a coup d'état at the French photographer's studio. In the fashion industry, models have a different agent for each city they work in. At this time I had ten.

"They're launching a new campaign, and they're looking for someone a little different who can stand out a bit. Cameron, you have just the sort of look that they're going for."

"That," I said, "is absolutely brilliant."

My girlfriend at the time was also my Paris agent, and she accompanied me on the flight to New York to meet with the Americans. Even though she wasn't helping me to find gigs in America, it was good to have her along to get perspective on the business side of things. The day after we arrived in New York, we headed down to the fashion district on Seventh Avenue and entered the building in which the company's offices were located.

"Malcolm will see you now," an assistant said to me from the door after we had been waiting in the lobby for a few minutes.

Malcolm was the casting agent, essentially in charge of deciding whom to hire for the label's various campaigns. I followed the assistant through the company's sleek hallways until I arrived at an office in the back corner overlooking the busy streets of the fashion district.

"Cameron," Malcolm said with a big smile as I walked through the door, "what an absolute pleasure." He got up from his desk and we shook hands, but he seemed to hold on for a moment before letting go. He was a few inches shorter than me, and I estimated he was somewhere in his midforties.

"It's a pleasure to meet you too," I said. He gestured to the chair in front of his desk as he took his seat again.

"So tell me what you've been up to lately."

"Well, I've been doing a lot of shows in Milan for Versace, Valentino, Dolce & Gabbana. You know, the usual."

"Right, right," he said.

"And I've been doing editorials for magazines like *Marie Claire, Vogue, Arena,* and *Elle.*"

"Right, right. Good, yes, I saw some of them, great stuff." He stared at me for a moment. "And who are your favorite photographers?"

"Well, I like Ellen Von Unwerth, who I have been working with a lot. Herb Ritz and Bruce Weber, of course."

"Right, right. Bruce is good." He continued to stare, his eyes drifting down to my chest and torso.

I started to get the feeling that it didn't really matter what I said because he kept checking me out and it didn't seem to be professional interest. This was a bit distracting, as I really wanted this interview to go well.

"Well, I feel really good about this. I think we can work together." He got up from behind his desk.

"That's . . . great!" I almost stammered. "Cool, very cool."

Malcolm walked me out as he asked me about my interests. I felt a little nervous, as if my mouth might say things my mind was not sure of, so I confined my answers to generalities like loving to travel and meeting new people. I didn't want to blow it. I was finally going to be in a major American campaign, and superstardom looked like it was within reach!

"Cameron, it's been a real pleasure," he said as he gave me another one of his lingering handshakes. We walked back out into the reception area.

"Who's that?" he asked as my girlfriend got up from the couch to greet me.

"That's my girlfriend," I said.

"Oh." He furrowed his brow. "Oh, yes. Your girlfriend."

"Um," I looked back at her, "it's cold outside, so, I guess I didn't want her to have to—"

"That's fine. We'll be in touch."

"How did it go?" my girlfriend asked as we got on the elevator.

"I think it went pretty good," I said, though something weird had just happened and I didn't know what it was.

The following day we were enjoying our afternoon when the phone rang. It was my New York agent.

"Cameron, what happened when you met with Malcolm?" she asked.

"Well, we talked for a bit about what I'd done and the photographers I liked. Why?"

"Did you say something to him about having a girlfriend?"

I recollected what we had talked about in my mind. "No, I don't think so. He saw her when she was waiting for me in the lobby, but they never spoke or anything. Is something wrong?"

"You didn't get the gig."

"Wh—what?"

"He told me that you shouldn't have brought your girlfriend there. He said he didn't want to give you the gig and that you shouldn't bother trying to work with his company ever again."

"Oh." I didn't know what else to say.

"I'm sorry, Cameron, I think he just got attached to the idea of you being single or something." She was making a very good effort to not keep the disappointment out of her own voice.

"Well, I'm sorry too," I said. "I didn't know that was going to be a problem."

And, that was that. I didn't get the gig. My girlfriend had heard my half of the conversation and didn't even ask what happened. Even if she hadn't heard it, she wouldn't have had to ask. The look on my face told her everything she needed to know. A door that had seemed wide open only seconds before now slammed in my face.

what is attachment?

Most of us, asked to define *attachment,* could probably come up with a slew of examples of things we can be attached to. "You know, like being attached to a piece of jewelry," one person might say. "My brother is really attached to his car," someone else is likely to declare. What is more difficult, though, is defining what attachment really is.

In trying to get the modeling gig at the American company, I was attached to the opportunity and potential benefits of starring in an advertising campaign of a major American design label. If I got that gig, then I would get a major boost in my goal of becoming as famous as the women who were emerging as the supermodels of the day. I acted as if my needs and desires would be satisfied only if I got the job. Not only that, but my quest to be the best led me to bring a competitive spirit to photo shoots, which led, as we saw, to other models getting replaced. Attachment, whether to an object, a person, an opportunity, or anything else, is wanting something in order to gratify the senses and satisfy the ego. In contrast, practicing detachment is the act of freeing oneself of sensual gratification for the sake of spiritual growth. This chapter will teach you what happens when we attach to something and how to practice detachment for the sake of living in joy and peace.

ATTACHMENT BEGINS WITH THE SENSES

What happens when you walk past a bakery and the smell of freshly baked rolls is wafting out? If you're like most people, you smell the baked goods, say to yourself, "Mmm . . . yummy rolls," and then duck into the bakery and buy some for immediate consumption and gratification. What happened here was that your senses fed you information about the rolls being nearby and edible, and then your imagination ran wild with possibilities of what they might taste like as you associated instant gratification with pleasure. On an intellectual and emotional level, you decided that you need to be a person in control. This experience demonstrates the onset of attachment, which begins with the senses.

Whether we receive information in the form of smells, sights, sounds, tastes, or touch, every experience in our lives is defined by how we respond to these many different stimuli. This is the importance of our senses. When we smell something wonderful cooking from inside a store and our senses are not under our control, we begin to crave that food. When we hear an ambulance's siren, we hope that no one we know is inside. When we see the look on our partner's face when she or he has been turned down for a job, we often feel disappointed on our loved one's behalf. If we feel particularly attached to the information delivered to us by our senses, we may eat the roll, call a friend or family member to make sure that person is okay, or criticize the employer that turned a partner down.

Where do these reactions come from? When our senses deliver information to the brain, our ego steps in and tells us that we want something. A conventional definition of *ego* is the consciousness of one's own identity or personality. Through the ego we focus on our outer surfaces and not on our inner selves. This part of the psyche mediates between our personalities and the realities around us; it shapes how we identify ourselves in response to the information coming through our senses. For our purposes, we can think of the ego as an ever-present mirage that seems real but that, once we have a spiritual practice, starts to fade so that the real self is revealed. Ego-based thought creates an identity based on status, control, and indulgence at the expense of finding real joy. It is the ego-based mentality that lies in the way of true happiness. Ego-based thought tells us that we need to have a certain logo on the side of our handbags to feel special, that we should value our jobs by our titles rather than by whether the work that we do is fulfilling, and that we must eat more luxurious foods to give us the sense that we are as elegant as the food is purported to be. It is the part of our minds focused on the outer world instead of on the inner guru. Whether or not we choose to indulge the ego on its mission to indulge our senses becomes the center of this practice.

ATTACHMENT LEADS TO FEAR

Why should it matter if our ego-based thoughts run free to dominate our actions? These thoughts make us feel that we need to look, act, and work a certain way because if we don't, then we will no longer have the opportunity to indulge our senses. When we have a lot of money, our egos make us feel that our lives will be miserable if we lose part or all of it. When we have access to the most exquisite foods, our ego-based thoughts make us believe and feel that we are not getting pleasure if our diets are bland and that we are not living fully if we don't indulge. If we don't have an impressive enough job, then we won't advance through life with the means to have more of whatever our ego-based thoughts have decided is important. If we are not in a relationship or even married, the ego-based thought gives us the wrong perception that we are not complete without another person beside us.

Imagining each of these possibilities leads, of course, to fear. When we allow ourselves to feel attached to something, we are setting ourselves up to want something or to feel that we're missing or lacking something. If we don't get what we want, we will be unhappy. Since none of us wants to be unhappy, we invest in fear and all the limitations that accompany it. Our ego-based minds use this fear as an incentive for us to consume more foods, work harder toward an impressive job title, buy more friends, and engage in more sensual pleasures. We do these things and they create imbalances in our bodies and minds. This is what most humans invest in on a daily basis.

The problem is, indulging our senses on behalf of obtaining things like status and control does not lead to true happiness. With this formula, happiness always depends on something or someone outside of us—on gratifying our ego-based thoughts. According to the traditions passed on to me by my teachers, this form of indulgence leads us to feel heavier and more weighted down by the material world. We might get a prestigious job title, but if we're attached to getting that title we'll just want to get an even more impressive title in the not-too-distant future. When we indulge in rich foods, our bodies tell us simply to get more of those foods as addiction sets in. When we decide that we want something and become attached to getting it, we are doing only one thing: *creating an opportunity to feel disappointed that we didn't get it.* Attachment leads to fear of this disappointment, which in turn creates our unhappiness and greater dis-appointment. It is a vicious cycle.

FEAR LEADS TO DESPERATION (NOT INSPIRATION)

What happens when we become fearful of not getting something? We act. We load ourselves up with food, wish ill will on co-workers, go on shopping sprees to buy more objects that we think will make us happy, or gossip and moan to our best friends about everything we want but don't have. When we attach ourselves to something or someone, we begin to feel the desperation and fear associated with not possessing it or them. We do things that hinder our growth and distract ourselves from knowing who we really are under the egos we have created and that we believe in so much.

The practice associated with freeing ourselves of our attachments, also known as detachment, helps us to find spiritual freedom. For our purposes, spiritual freedom is defined as living in a fully realized state beyond material, mental, and emotional limitations. The practice out-lined in this book centers on working toward this more awakened way of life, and those who commit to this path make decisions and take action with the intention of being true to their deepest selves. When these decisions and actions come from this place of spiritual realization, our progress through life becomes the product of inspiration rather than desperation.

In the story at the beginning of this chapter, I was very attached to getting the American designer job. Even though the man interviewing me seemed to have additional interests beyond filling the spot in the ad campaign, I was still willing to accommodate his obvious stares and was nervous about talking to him about something as simple as my general interests. My ego-based thoughts told me that my life might be empty without this job, and I was fearful of such a thing. Because of this fear, I wasn't really myself and pandered to someone who clearly had dubi-ous intentions.

When we make decisions from a truthful and detached place, our ac-tions are full of energy and inspiration. In the following section we'll explore what it means to be detached from something and how to incor-porate detachment into our practice and our lives.

what is detachment?

Theresa was attached to her boyfriend. She felt she needed him even though he often drank alcohol and as a result didn't make himself emotionally available to her. When she came to me, she was incapable of sitting still for more than a couple of seconds, and she seemed to suffer from a complete lack of confidence. She told me that she would often try to initiate activities for them to do together, only to be turned down by him in favor of sitting around the house with that night's drink of choice. If he did want to go out, it was usually with a couple of his buddies, and they simply sat around drinking together. When I asked her why she stayed with him, she told me that they had been together for years and she couldn't imagine herself being with anyone else.

Theresa was exhibiting classic behaviors of attachment to her boyfriend. Even though she felt that he was not treating her well, their time together seemed to have taught her that she would not be desirable to another man. She stayed with him out of fear of losing what they had shared and because being with him was better than not being with anyone at all. I worked with Theresa on certain breathing exercises with the intention of balancing male and female energy and taught her yoga postures that soothed her and helped her to build enough confidence to let go of her attached feelings. Through these practices she was able to observe herself in this relationship and could see that there were fundamental problems to be dealt with. Because she had worked to build her confidence and shift her intentions, she was able to engage her boyfriend in a dialogue about their relationship. He recognized that her request for a dialogue was now rooted not in neediness but in maturity and stability and that she no longer feared losing him.

This story demonstrates how we can use our practice to free ourselves of our attachments. To detach from her relationship, Theresa had to observe the role her own ego was playing in keeping her lost in her fears ("What if I never find someone else?"). If, however, she had gone in the opposite direction, suddenly throwing her hands up and quitting the relationship without any reflection, she would have been denying herself an opportunity to investigate what had compelled her to stay in the relationship for as long as she had. This would have been succumbing to a different fear ("What if I get stuck in this relationship forever?").

Developing the kind of awareness that was required of Theresa, as you might imagine, can be a challenge—especially for something as significant as a romantic relationship. How do we know if, when we decide to let go of something, we're really just detaching and not simply denying ourselves an opportunity to enjoy ourselves? If we are attached to something, we become fearful of not having it. We think we must get a certain amount of it, by a certain time, or with certain conditions. If, however, we succeed in becoming detached, we acknowledge the basic truth that everything in life has its moment, and if we don't eat a certain food, get a certain job, or have a certain relationship, there's a better time for it to happen—or it might not have to happen at all.

Let me repeat that: if we are detached from something that doesn't take place, we understand and believe that there's a better time for it to happen or that it is not meant for our journey at this moment.

As I mentioned above, Theresa became aware of the truth of her relationship. She understood that while it would be good for her relationship to work out, not being in it would in no way mean the end of her happiness. She shifted her intention to live as an example and make their life together as good as she possibly could, and it was no surprise when she told me months after we had begun working together that her boyfriend hardly ever drank, they spent several enjoyable nights a week together, they had both lost weight, and that they were getting married the following year. Theresa had succeeded in detaching from her situation, and if she had denied herself an opportunity to explore herself in the relationship, she never would have found the happiness she did.

Not all situations turn out this way. Many people decide to move on, as their partners do not want to change or advance in life. Either way, because we put our attention first on happiness and not on the other person as the source of that happiness, we are content with our lives and choices. The only way to truly help others change for the better is by changing our own ways for others to see.

how to practice detachment

There are as many opportunities to attach ourselves to something as there are experiences in a lifetime. Each experience presents us with the possibility of loss. Having the potential to lose so many things not only demonstrates why fear has come to be such a significant factor in the decisions we make, but it also shows the potential benefit of practicing detachment. If we practice detachment in our day-to-day lives, then we can free ourselves of fearing unhappiness and loss.

The challenge, of course, is to not feel overwhelmed by the many different moments that we have the potential of attaching ourselves to. If I were to simply say to you, "Go now, live without fear, and detach yourself from everything that happens in your life," you'd probably have no idea where to begin. Detachment is a significant and ambitious practice, but this final section of the chapter will outline five basic areas of your life in which you can begin to do the work. Given the diverse and dynamic nature of the human experience, we could likely fill up several books with many more than five ways of beginning this practice. What follows, though, will give you a start.

GOODS AND OBJECTS

Whether we crave a certain food or drink, consume controlled substances, collect trinkets, or own an heirloom of significant sentimental value, most of us can relate in some way to being attached to physical goods and objects. Our attachment to these things stems from a fear that without a certain level of abundance and physical gratification, we will not live a long and prosperous life. The irony of this, of course, is that many of us wind up shortening our lives because of disease associated with what we put into our bodies and the stress of getting too much or not enough of what we want.

Detachment, as noted above, involves acknowledging the likelihood that there may be a better time to get what we want or that it is more beneficial that we don't have it at all. Practicing detachment from goods and objects, as with all of the detachment practices described below, is an extension of this idea. It simply requires us to tell ourselves that something that we're fearful of not having may come into our lives at a different and more appropriate time. Freshly baked rolls will be available tomorrow, another trinket might make us forget the trinkets we already have, and we could always commission another object to commemorate the person who gave us the heirloom—if something were to ever happen to the heirloom itself. A question to contemplate is: Why does a material object take the place of the memories of the person who gave it to us? The exercise above can help you in beginning to detach from physical things.

roll over next week

A classic example of feeling attached to something physical is smelling a freshly baked or cooked food item and wanting to have it. In this exercise, take a walk past a bakery, favorite restaurant, or shop or somewhere that is always tempting you to indulge your sense of taste, and instead of satisfying that urge, pamper your other senses, like smell and sight. Don't, however, let go to the point of drooling—that can be embarrassing. Then leave without buying, consuming, or staying too long. Note the day and time that you had this experience, and then come back exactly a week later to enjoy a little more.

The idea of this exercise is to help you to train your mind not to depend on instant gratification of the senses but instead to accept that there will be another opportunity in the future to consume your object of desire. You don't need instant physical gratification. The intention here is to delay gratification of your senses in order to give yourself something to reflect on instead of feeling the usual stress and determination to get what you want. When you do return a week later, indulge in a moderate and small way, but consider if your needs are really needs or are merely uncontrolled wants. If you don't even feel the need to engage in the moment after the week is up, then you've completely succeeded in detaching yourself from the item. This is how we build willpower, which I'll discuss in the next chapter.

If you are a fan of shopping and tend to enter stores to make impulsive purchases, then this exercise can be applied in a similar way. The next time you're walking past a store that usually tempts you to go in and buy something, like an article of clothing, shoes, or jewelry, take a moment to observe that desire, and try to commit yourself to not buying the object until a later time. If, a couple of weeks later, you're walking by and don't feel compelled to buy the object, then you've not only detached from it but you probably didn't need it in the first place.

EXPERIENCES

We live in a culture that seeks pleasure. We love to go to the beach, go out to eat with friends, travel, and enjoy all sorts of other ways of entertaining ourselves. What happens, though, when we find out that our trip is canceled or someone changed the plans? It is easy to become attached to activities we think we will have fun doing and hard not to feel disappointed when they don't work out. Ego-based thought tells us that we won't be happy if we don't fill our lives with entertaining experiences, and

silent lunch

When we meet a friend or family member for lunch, we likely have many things to talk about. Sometimes we ask a friend for advice about a challenging situation, but more often we fill up the experience with chatter because we are afraid of not having anything interesting to say or of feeling awkward in the silence. Our friend, in turn, has plenty of things to chat about as well. This kind of idle conversation perpetuates useless interactions instead of fulfilling a specific purpose.

Ask a friend or family member out to lunch. Commit yourself to talking very little and instead just enjoying your friend's company and listening to what she or he has to say. When you've both been seated, allow your friend to talk as much as desired, and if your friend falls silent, observe yourself in this silence. The practice is to overcome your fear of not feeling interesting and to detach yourself from needing to fill the time up with meaningless chatter.

When doing this exercise, I suggest you wait until the end of the lunch to reveal to your friend what you were doing. If you announce it beforehand, the situation will become unnatural. If your friend comments during lunch on how you seem different or are acting strangely, resist the urge to confess what you're doing. Instead, reply that you want to listen more and that you are very interested in what she or he is talking about. When you do tell your friend what you have been doing, consider adding some reassurance that you chose to do the exercise out of a real desire to enjoy your friend's company in this new and different way.

we become fearful of living out the rest of our lives in a bland, unpleasant stupor. A student of mine once told me that he was afraid to meditate because he thought his life would become boring. Ironically, he was not very fond of the life he was currently living.

When we practice detachment from experiences, we are training ourselves to know that while one experience may not pan out like we would like, another one is around the corner. Our work is to allow ourselves to enjoy an experience when it finds its way to us and to let go of the experiences that either aren't enjoyable or simply aren't meant to be. If we learn to accept and adapt to what comes, then that experience becomes the right one for us in the moment and prepares us for the next experience or opportunity to come.

OPPORTUNITY

What happens when we hear or see a job description that we feel is absolutely perfect for us? What happens when we send creative writing or other material out to someone who can publish the work? What happened when we auditioned for the lead in the school play during our sophomore year in high school even though the seniors were always the ones who got the leads? If we are attached to these or other opportunities, we picture ourselves getting the job or contract or part, we imagine what it will feel like to bask in the glory of that accomplishment, and then we feel absolutely crushed if we don't get it. Attaching ourselves to an opportunity for growth or advancement in something is a classic and common habit. We decide something must go a certain way, and when it doesn't happen in that way we are disappointed and fearful of never having an opportunity like that again.

Detaching ourselves from an opportunity can be a difficult thing to do, especially if attaining that opportunity will deliver a significant boost in our ability to make a living. I might have been disappointed by not getting

football without sides

One experience that many of us can relate to is getting together with a group of friends and watching a football game or another sporting event. Hot wings and pizza are delivered, bottles of beer are passed around, and most if not all of this food and drink is finished off by the end of the game. What is often a significant part of this experience, though, is an intense desire for one team to beat the other.

The exercise is to practice detachment from your preferred team winning and instead to simply watch the game as an exciting contest in and of itself. Rather than investing your energy into one side winning, spend the time observing the extent of the players' ability, whether or not you find each of the team's plays reflects good decisions by the coaches, and which team you feel is playing a better game. Once the game is over, notice if you've changed any of your other behaviors. Have you eaten less food? Do you feel less drained from the experience? Have you had a better time overall? Are you less nervous?

While it's likely that you'll want to go back to rooting for your team the following week, notice if practicing this exercise has any sort of trickle-down effect on your experiences over time.

the American campaign, but if I had been practicing back then I would have been able to center myself on the idea that another opportunity to work on a similar advertising campaign might present itself shortly. Instead, I felt devastated. Detachment from an opportunity requires us to accept that if we don't get something we've pursued, it is simply what nature has intended for us.

The next time a seemingly perfect opportunity presents itself, consider at least three other opportunities that would be even more beneficial, and set your intention to pursue one of them if this first opportunity doesn't pan out.

OPINIONS

We love our opinions. We love having them. We might declare that a movie we just saw is the worst movie ever made, and we might believe it. Yet just because we have made this declaration, it does not mean our opinion is true. When we form an opinion such as this, we can become vehemently attached to it and will go to any length to defend it.

To understand what it feels like to be attached to an opinion, all you have to do is think of the last time you disagreed with somebody. You stated your opinion then waited for a retort. Do you remember the satisfaction you felt when the other person had no good comeback? We experience a fear of being wrong, and this fear forms the basis of a lot of arguments, debates, disagreements, and other heated discussions that blow up in our faces and even end relationships. If we're wrong, then surely we are less worthy as human beings, right? Of course, the answer is no.

Removing the ego from a difference of opinion with another person is difficult because we hold on to the notion that we are right. Opinions are self-formed and really have little or nothing to do with what is objectively true, which is why they cause so much discord among people. If we can simply observe the other person's words and not compare them to ours, then we are taking the first step toward detachment from opinions and control. Detachment does not, however, mean that we agree with the other person's opinions or point of view; it means only that we're not going to allow the difference in perspectives to create fear in us. This allows us to listen without attachment to other people's opinions as well as our own.

listen to a difference of opinion

In the previous chapter on violence, you practiced watching an irritating personality on television and limiting yourself to observing details unrelated to what the person was saying, such as what the person was wearing or the simple fact that the person was talking. That exercise is excellent for developing detachment as well. For the sake of focusing specifically on practicing detachment from opinions, this exercise centers on observing what a live person is actually saying.

Sit or stand facing a friend or family member while he or she presents an opinion that differs from your own. That person might believe in a different religion, support a different political party, or simply feel that one recipe for chocolate chip cookies is better than the one that you consider the best. Whatever the case, your friend or relative explains why she or he is right. As your friend begins talking, note to yourself one opinion being expressed, and say to yourself, "He or she feels that _____." It's not necessary to think about how your opinion is different from your friend's, only to acknowledge that this person feels a certain way. Have this person talk for only a minute at first, and if she or he is willing to practice this exercise with you again, begin to lengthen the amount of time the person talks by minute-long increments. In this practice, detachment does not mean ignoring others; rather, it means giving someone your full attention without giving away your emotions or intellect.

Given how sensitive people can be about their opinions and how easily they can become defensive, it is important to do this exercise with someone you trust and also to explain ahead of time why you're doing it in the first place. Consider having the person read the description of this exercise to better understand your intentions, and reiterate that you've chosen this person because of your trust in him or her to be able to help you grow.

RELATIONSHIPS

Anyone who has ever been broken up with, divorced, ended a friendship, or lost a loved one knows how much emotional pain can emerge from an ended or troubled relationship. More to the point, those of us who do not have anyone special in our lives can feel an intense sense of emptiness as well. The connection we feel to another person may well be one of the strongest attachments we experience in life, as was evidenced by my client Theresa's story. Given the powerful nature of this connection, there is

write a letter

Though there are many ways to explore our attachments in relationships, I'd like to offer a very simple exercise as a first step. Because your practice in this area affects other people, it's particularly important that you are sensitive to other people's needs.

Choose one person you normally see or talk to on the phone at least a few times a week—a friend, sibling, parent, or someone else you feel close to and have a solid relationship with. The task is to not talk to this person for a week and instead to write him or her a letter—not an e-mail, a letter. If the person does not receive the letter by the end of the week, that's okay. The idea is to take some time to observe yourself in this week of silence and also to use the very personal act of writing a letter to explore your relationship with this person. By not having your regular conversations, you allow this other person to live her or his life separate from you, and you use the one-sided act of writing the letter as a way to separate your ego from how and if the other person responds.

As in the previous exercise, be sure to tell your friend why you are doing this and to make sure the person knows that you do not intend to create distance but simply want to observe your relationship and the degree of attachment you have. Also be sure to invite your friend to ask questions, and answer them as best as you can.

likewise a significant potential to fear the loss of a relationship or to feel rejected when another person doesn't share an interest in pursuing one.

The sensitivity of relationships makes the act of becoming detached from them a delicate process. While it may seem like detachment from a person is equivalent to not caring about them, I encourage you to recognize this practice as simply letting the person be who she or he is separate from what our ego-based thought wants that person to be. Imagine what would happen if a mother attached herself to her children when they're first born and never let them grow up to become independent people. The children would likely feel smothered and controlled and would become imbalanced in their own relationships. At the beginning stages of this practice, we have an opportunity to observe ourselves in our relationships with others and to work toward letting go of unfulfilled fantasies and other ideas of what we think those relationships should be.

As you can see, there are many different ways we can practice detachment. Fear is a very powerful emotion for many of us, and because of this, detachment will be one of the most difficult parts of our practice. I hope, though, that you make it a central part of your path toward happiness and that your silent example invites others to do the same. The act of detachment can and will help you to live a life of fearlessness and joy.

. . .

True to Malcolm's word, I never did work for his company. While I wasn't aware of detachment all those years ago in my early twenties, I did have a sense that other things were coming my way. Within a month of the disastrous meeting with Malcolm, I received another phone call.

"Cameron," my agent in New York said, "Guess would like to see you."

"I don't know," I said. "Who?"

"No," she laughed. "Guess. The American jeans label. They'd like to see you."

"Oh," I said. "Oh! Right! That's good news."

"The meeting is in three days. You'll be able to take care of your ticket?"

"I've got the frequent flyer miles," I said. "I've been traveling to New York a lot lately."

"Right. Best not to bring your girlfriend to the building this time."

"What girlfriend?" I laughed. That certainly wasn't going to be a problem.

A week later I got the call that the Guess jeans job was mine. It would last for the next two years. A certain Material Girl would see that campaign and tell her manager to hire me for her next video.

The course of events that followed was exactly what was meant to be, and anything else would have been a distraction.

This is, ultimately, what nature intends for all of us.

fill in the blank

The act of practicing detachment is the immediate predecessor to the practice outlined in the following chapter. To establish a more solid understanding of this relationship, prac-tice at least two or three of the five exercises provided in this chapter before moving on to chapter 5.

5 letting go of excess

knowing when enough is enough
(or the perfect amount)

N 1992 I SAW A MAN backstage at a Jean Paul Gaultier show making a group of people laugh. His name was Benjamin, and he was speaking to a bunch of models.

"How many models does it take to screw in a lightbulb?" Benjamin asked his audience.

"How many?" asked the young woman closest to him.

"Four," Benjamin said. "One to screw it in and three to say, 'You look *fabulous* doing that.'"

The models all cracked up. His humor was infectious. Benjamin was a friendly, funny, and incredibly attractive boy with a smile gaining more and more attention from the clients, and it was common to see him at the center of attention. He just seemed happy to be working in Paris.

I had been in the fashion industry for several years and had noticed Benjamin here and there as we worked the same shows. My musician friend Jessie had noticed him as well. She developed a little crush.

"Cam," she said, "the next time you run into him, invite him to party."

"He's a party on his own," I replied.

While Benjamin was known by day for his engaging personality, by night he was known as a heavy drinker. Jessie was too, which I was sure was part of the reason she was drawn to him. I had enjoyed my fair share of substance use on occasion, but my limits were much lower than these two party professionals. My most indulgent experience to date had been going to a party in a hotel room, taking half a hit of ecstasy, and maybe smoking a joint. The drugs might have made my companions rampantly horny, but they inspired me simply to sit by the bathroom and comment on how enchanted people looked while they entered and left the toilet.

About six months after the Gaultier show, I ran into Benjamin at my agency's office in New York. He recognized me, and while my friend Jessie's plea for his company rang in my ears, I didn't have to instigate anything.

"You busy tonight?" Benjamin asked with his increasingly famous smile. "Wanna hang out?"

"Of course," I replied. "I'll ask my friend Jessie to hang as well."

They both arrived at my apartment in Hell's Kitchen at about eight in the evening. Benjamin brought two bottles of Jack Daniels and two bottles of Coke, and we got started right away.

"You know, Cameron, you're really nursing that drink," Benjamin said as he poured his second.

"Yeah, Cam," Jessie said, "you have to work tomorrow?"

I looked down at my glass, which was still two-thirds full.

"Yeah, well, you know." I took a sip. "I don't know that I could keep up with you guys."

Jessie and Benjamin shared a knowing look.

"What if you tried a little harder?" Benjamin asked, his smile breaking out.

"What if I tried what a little harder?"

"What if you tried matching us drink for drink?" Benjamin said. "We would have a blast, man. Besides, drinking works up an appetite."

"Ooh," Jessie said, "there's a new restaurant that's opened up just around the corner on Ninth Avenue!"

I looked at them. They might have been very excited about this idea, but I wasn't sure it was something I could do. I also knew, however, that this was simply one of the things that fast-paced people did as part of the culture of being, in this case, models.

"All right," I said, "I'll play along. For you guys."

So it began. I caught up with Benjamin's second Jack and Coke within a few minutes and started on my third.

"It's not that you have to be drunk to have a good time," Benjamin said after he swigged the rest of his fourth drink and started on his fifth, "but it definitely helps." I think I agreed as I finished my fourth as well, but I was too distracted with how the Coke label started to read like "Crack." After several minutes, I chalked it up to a change in the soda company's formula.

Somewhere around drink six we decided that we were hungry, and they walked while I hovered over to Ninth Avenue. We didn't make it to the restaurant Jessie wanted to go to because she couldn't remember where it was. I wondered if the place had ever existed at all. Benjamin decided he wanted to find a place with good Indian food. He declared our search a success when we found a Spanish restaurant with excellent paella. This made sense to us because after that many Jack and Cokes, Spain and India are basically the same country. I had some sort of food, but I was too distracted with trying to get my lemon out of my third beer to remember what I ate.

I'm pretty sure we went to a pool hall after dinner, as I have a vague memory of trying to hit a cue ball with a stick and not knowing the difference between the balls that were real and those that weren't. Benjamin must have won the game we were playing, for he was using the cue stick as if it were a pole at a strip club. I was too distracted by the fear of what would happen if he started taking his clothes off to care about the game's outcome. I had stopped drinking shortly after our arrival at the hall, and Jessie must have too. Benjamin continued drinking until we left.

An image of being pushed into a cab seems to be in there somewhere, as was not getting home until 6:00 or 9:00 (the numbers kept spinning) the following morning. Bewildered, drained, and horribly, horribly drunk, I finally wandered to bed. As soon as my head found the pillow, I was out cold.

what is excess?

In our culture it has become acceptable for us to feel an unnatural amount of pain, discomfort, and disease as we get older. It is standard for men to develop issues with their prostate or heart and typical for women to suffer through PMS, tumors, and menopause. Recent findings made by the National Health Interview Survey stated that nearly 10 percent of us experience chronic lower back pain, a number that has increased nearly threefold since the early 1990s. We no longer wonder if we will ever get cancer and instead are resigned to asking when and what type. What ancient teachings show us, however, is that all of these obstacles are simply the result of our behaviors—behaviors that can, ultimately, be modified to eliminate these problems.

Many of us have more than one story of excess. Eating too much food for Christmas dinner leaves us on the couch with a bloated, gassy feeling for the few minutes we maintain consciousness before passing out. Smoking cigarettes causes us to cough up all sorts of unpleasant things, and partaking in continual sexual activities can leave us feeling drained and exhausted. Excessive alcohol consumption, as the above story shows, causes us to moan our way through the early morning hours and makes us wish we'd never had the evening we had—if we can even remember that it happened in the first place.

We often give ourselves permission to have that big meal because it's a special holiday or weekend, and many of us have drunk to the point of puking. What we're concerned about in the context of this practice, however, is not just how we put ourselves through misery in specific, isolated incidents but how our daily habits and routines lead to health problems like the ones noted above. *Excess* is defined as any behavior that stops the body and mind from functioning in a natural way. The excessive behaviors we'll explore in this chapter may include the extreme examples from above, but they primarily focus on behaviors that are generally accepted as normal and appropriate.

excess stems from attachment

In the previous chapter we learned that much of what happens to us in our lives is defined by our attachments. I became very attached to becoming the best and most successful model in the industry and, by feeling cool and untouchable in my trendy Ray Petri look, brought an elitist attitude to work that was not productive to everyone. Our attachments, as the chapter stated, are born from our existence in the material world and stem from thoughts that breed selfish actions. These attachments cause us to crave certain experiences that we think will help us gratify our egos, which leads us to take more and more of those kinds of actions to benefit ourselves. Eventually we take so many of these actions on behalf of our egos that we push our bodies and minds completely out of balance. These various ego-based actions are, ultimately, excessive behaviors that lead to our suffering.

Let us look at my drinking story as an example. As I've explained, I was attached to the fashion industry in the late 1980s and early 1990s. My sense of self-worth was dependent upon my status in the industry and whether or not I worked for the best labels, had the right friends, and could afford more than one living space. I wasn't really into drinking and experimenting with substances, yet I was willing to spend an evening with a guy I didn't know very well and imbibe drink after drink after drink. As often happens with such behaviors, I was barely functioning by the end of the experience. I was so attached to Benjamin's infectious energy of letting go in the moment that I was willing to join in excessive drinking for the sake of being accepted and feeling a buzz. Had I been more detached from these ideas of success and popularity, then I wouldn't have felt the need to indulge in excess. I would have spared myself a lot of discomfort and pain.

indulging in excess

To live in balance, we need a few basic staples such as food, water, and shelter. Some of us need more of certain items than others, like a marathon runner requiring greater amounts of sustenance than a person who is bedridden. Supporting our ability to live requires us to eat a certain amount, think a certain amount, and participate in a certain amount of physical or mental activity. Any other actions we take beyond the satisfaction of our basic needs become excessive.

When we take proper actions to live, we feel an ease of comfort and balance in our bodies and minds. When we engage in actions that are excessive, however, the body defends itself. Thinking too much can lead to a condition like insomnia or hypertension. Eating too much or too quickly can lead to constipation, indigestion, flatulence, or headaches. Regardless of how we exhibit excessive behaviors, the body and mind will have to invest energy in restoring balance, which will in turn create discomfort and pain. Below is a list of the different ways that we may indulge in excess and what happens when the body's need to defend itself against such excesses creates disharmony and imbalance. You will recognize several of these examples from chapter 1.

Food: Eating excessive amounts of food not only can lead to obesity, but it will also tax the body's ability to heal itself and properly circulate energy, thus leading to above-mentioned conditions such as constipation and headaches.

Alcohol: Consuming alcohol will require the body to purge itself of toxins more than is necessary. It therefore uses physical resources that would otherwise be directed toward maintaining basic health and is of absolutely no use to the system.

Smoking and drugs: Any form of stimulation through drugs and other controlled substances creates a dependence on chemicals that the body doesn't produce naturally. Because the substances are foreign to our bodies, our systems invest valuable energy in their removal.

Fitness: Fitness is born from our ego-based thoughts and is not the same thing as health. Those who train excessively to attain a state of fitness can experience a chronic sense of fatigue, inflammation in the muscles and connective tissues, and a disabled immune system.

Sex: Practicing excessive amounts of sexual activity will lead to exhaustion, diminished vitality, sexual dysfunction, and the sapping of life.

Money and possessions: Investing an excessive amount of energy in earning money for the sake of status and accumulation can create aggression and frustration, which then lead to stress.

Work and success: Recall Michael in chapter 1, the manager and editor of national magazines who pursued success so relentlessly that he developed allergies, indigestion, and bad sleep. Those who overwork in the way that Michael did will likely cause themselves stress to the point of creating illness and weakness in the body.

Relationships: When we're emotionally attached to our friends and families to an excessive degree, we create roles for them that they are unlikely to ever be able to fulfill. We risk sabotaging those relationships when we challenge our loved ones for not fulfilling our needs.

Thinking: An excessive amount of thinking leads to headaches, stress, and anxiety, which in turn lead to disease.

Talking: An excessive amount of verbalizing cuts our breathing to a point that we start to expire, rather than inspire, our bodies and minds. It also adds to other people's stress.

You may have noticed that I rarely provide specific parameters for determining how much of any one thing is excessive. This is for good reason:

letting go of excess

the process of being guided by your inner guru involves observing your own life to determine how much of any one thing is excessive. Generally, however, we can follow certain guidelines for some of the behaviors. We're eating too much if we're becoming heavy or overweight, we're thinking too much if we get constant headaches, and so forth. Throughout the remainder of the chapter, we'll explore how you can use the guru in you to train yourself to eliminate disease in your body by changing excessive behaviors.

willpower: that ever-elusive force

Susan was a client of mine who suffered from morbid obesity. At thirty-five, she was on antidepressants, had mentally abusive relationships including a boyfriend who lived with another woman (yes, you read that right), and couldn't focus on one thing for more than twenty seconds. Susan was the embodiment of dysfunction through excess, as she ate continuously, smoked twenty-five cigarettes a day, and drank five espressos daily.

I worked with Susan to acknowledge the root cause of her destructive lifestyle and to see that these behaviors weren't serving her. The process helped her free herself of her excessive practices. We started with discussions intended to help her bring awareness to the cause of her frustrations. We determined that she was attracted to anyone and anything that kept her in a negative cycle, and with this information we set a routine that required her to do the opposite of what she would have normally chosen. As she was too stiff and large for practicing yoga postures, I taught her basic breathing exercises that required little movement. I recommended that she stop taking the antidepressants, suggested that she eat only once a day at 2:00 p.m., and replaced the espresso with herbal concoctions. At the beginning of our time together, we worked together to shift her intention toward not indulging in excess, and once we started working she no longer felt hungry all the time, reduced her smoking, and chose to eat smaller portions when she did eat. While she had spent many years suffering through spotty sleep from 1:00 a.m. to 9:00 a.m., she was able to go to bed at 10:00 p.m. and wake up feeling rested at 7:00 a.m.

In addition to modifying her habits, we worked out how her frustrations were feeding her excesses. As a result, this transformation happened in an astonishingly short period of time—just two days.

Now, most people can appreciate the extent and the significance of the change in Susan's lifestyle. As she was dealing with so many different issues, it was remarkable that she was able to restore so much balance to her body in such a short amount of time. However, it's also likely that every person who appreciates this change will also say something like, "Well sure, if I had someone like Yogi Cameron working with me for two days straight, I'd be able to remove excess from my lifestyle like that as well." Indeed, most of us could. This is because I played a very specific role when working with Susan. My knowledge, focus, and overall energy provided a significant source of motivation for Susan not to sneak a late-night snack, break out the cigarettes, or take just three little sips of espresso. In short, I was Susan's source of willpower.

Willpower, or the discipline to follow through on an intention, is the only tool we have for overcoming our excessive practices. I'm sure that my message would be much more appealing right now if I said that excess can be resolved through taking a pill three times a day or by investing in a new, state-of-the-art self-help kit (as seen on TV for only $499.95). This is not, in fact, the case. If you remove excess from your life through the process outlined below, you are endeavoring to find your own sense of truth and to discover your basic purpose. This process becomes, in essence, your spiritual practice. Whether you pursue the plan outlined in this book or follow someone else's program, it's tremendously important to understand one thing: it is your willpower to practice and only your willpower to practice that will define your change. If we worked together, I could help get you started, but only you can completely make the change you want. Without the actual action of practice, nothing can be attained.

Susan, despite all of the very real changes that took place in her life in the short time we had together, did not continue with her practice. I provided a series of exercises that she could use to develop her willpower, but once I left her home she regressed back to her old habits, as it was the easier path to take. Her abusive boyfriend did not think very highly of Susan taking control of her life, as she seemed to be doing, and convinced her to not have me back. Had she followed through, even for several weeks, she would have given herself a much greater chance of long-term change and attracted a better-mannered man into her life.

how to build your willpower

Susan's story, unfortunately, is much more common than the alternative of people finding a path toward happiness and having the willpower to stick to it. We become attached to our pursuit of pleasure and finding the easier way out. Bodies continue to be taxed with excessive habits, minds continue to be burdened with excessive thoughts, and because people set intentions that don't include the benefit of those around them, they rarely find the support they need from others to continue on their way. I don't want this for you, and this section outlines how to build your willpower so that your intentions can manifest as a consistent and inspired part of your new and better life. However, for your practice to mature, you'll need to dedicate some time to it.

Building your willpower is similar to building muscle in your body or advancing through different levels of training. When starting to ride a bike, you do not try to climb the steepest mountain but start by riding up smaller hills to first practice resistance training. You start with the shorter distances and work your way up to the longer ones. When you participate in a yoga class for the first time, you take an introductory class that teaches you the basics, and as your body naturally opens up, you eventually proceed to the more advanced classes. If you pursue a martial art, you start training as a white belt and advance to a black belt. This is also true for building willpower.

Most of us who begin a practice such as the one outlined in this book do not have particularly developed willpower. If we do any sort of self-improvement practice like exercise or diet, it's usually only for a few days a week or in short-lived phases. Practicing the removal of excessive behaviors, though, is a daily routine. Every one of us can pick at least one or two items from the above list of behaviors that challenge us every day. The practice is to simply acknowledge those challenges and will ourselves to overcome them by setting our intention from the beginning and detaching ourselves from the result. As noted earlier in the chapter, when we overcome these excessive behaviors, we create a greater opportunity to live in balance.

How, though, do we build the muscles to make this happen? The following three techniques will help you go from the white belt, so to speak, to the black.

WILLPOWER BEGINS WITH DISTRACTION

Let's say you're a person who loves a rich dessert after dinner each night, and even though you go to bed feeling sluggish and wasted an hour later, dessert is one of your favorite times of day. You know that you shouldn't eat such decadent foods every night, but you crave them all the same. What would happen if one evening after dinner you were deciding what dessert to have and the phone rang with a call from your brother-in-law saying that your sister had just had her baby? After the initial screaming and whooping, you'd probably spend a few minutes asking about the baby's weight and health, and you might probe your brother-in-law for stories about how your sister's labor went. For the twenty or thirty minutes that you were learning about your new niece or nephew, it's likely that you would no longer be thinking about dessert. Your standard routine was disrupted because you experienced a diversion of thought.

The first step of developing your willpower and removing excess from your life is to create a positive distraction for yourself. As in the above example, when we're distracted from thinking about one thing, we're focusing on another thought that is more worthy of our immediate attention. Learning of a new baby in the family can distract us from whatever we're doing, but we can't count on receiving a call like that every day—and certainly not at the exact moment that we need to abstain from an excessive behavior. Instead, we begin to build our willpower muscles when we create some sort of activity to focus on at whatever time we need to abstain from a behavior. If you always go for a rich dessert after your meal, then perhaps you can make a phone call, wash the car, read a book, or take up a hobby that is good for both the mind and body. If you're inclined to drink alcohol to unwind from a tough day at work, then perhaps you can ask a roommate or neighbor to join you for herbal tea in the dining room, and you can talk to them about your day or discuss new habits for bettering your lives. Distract yourself with some yoga postures as presented later in the book, or assist someone who needs a helping hand. Your redirection of energy needs to be spent on a useful activity, and when you effectively distract yourself from an excessive behavior for even a few minutes, you're laying the groundwork to free yourself from that habit for good.

distract yourself

To create a distraction for yourself, simply choose an activity to do as an alternative to an excessive behavior at the time of day when you find yourself most prone to indulging. Once you've thought of an activity, ask yourself if it is an accurate reflection of your intention and if it will be useful in your life. It is sometimes a challenge, of course, to think of an activity, so below are some suggestions.

- **Excessive eating:** Reading spiritual material, going for a walk, having inspiring conversation with a positive person, journaling, completing puzzles, playing games with friends or family, e-mailing, playing sports, helping someone, taking the dog for a walk, or just going outside.

- **Excessive drinking:** Talking with a friend or family member over herbal tea, chatting with someone on the phone, finding a spiritual practice like yoga, helping someone with a specific task.

- **Smoking and drugs:** Breathing exercises as described in chapter 7.

- **Excessive exercise:** Yoga postures as described in chapter 6.

- **Excessive sex:** Postures as described in chapter 6.

- **Excessive acquisition of money and possessions:** Taking long walks, volunteering at homeless shelters, and other activities that require no money.

- **Excessive amounts of work:** Sharing a simple meal with someone without the company of your Blackberry and engaging in other activities that foster outside-of-work connections with other people—which will benefit them as well.

- **Excessive dependence on others:** Writing letters to people whom you usually see or speak with on a regular basis, sitting alone in silence for one hour a day in contemplation, helping someone.

- **Excessive thinking:** Concentration and sitting exercises as described in chapter 9.

It is possible, as Susan did, to work on all behaviors at the same time. Susan, however, had the advantage of someone staying in her home to help distract her from her behaviors, and since you don't have this, it is advised to try implementing only one distraction for one excessive behavior at a time. The key to success is repetition.

WILLPOWER AND QUANTITY

Many of the ways we indulge in excess involve quantity. We might eat too much food, drink too much alcohol, talk too much, think too much, or spend too much money. Though many of us have tried to control these habits by eliminating or curbing our actions, the philosophy of gradually building willpower suggests that we should do it a small amount at a time.

To begin building willpower, start with making a small change. Rather than eliminating all junk food from your snacking routine, estimate how much you typically eat for a particular snack, and serve yourself only three-quarters of that amount for one or two weeks. Rather than stopping money expenditures completely, take two-thirds of the amount you typically spend, and place the rest in a drawer. This practice is to show you from the start how much power you have over your actions. Once the mind is focused, you will demonstrate to yourself that you can happily live without these excesses. Regulating the quantity of an excessive behavior, but only incrementally, provides you with a basic tool for building your willpower muscles.

WILLPOWER AND TIME

We can also build our willpower through experimenting with duration of time. We may notice that our excessive behaviors usually are out of balance with respect to time; we may eat late at night, eat too quickly, spend too many hours of the day lost in thought, or work later than everyone else in the office. One way to build our willpower is to reshape how much or how little time we spend indulging in an excessive behavior. Just as in working with quantity, we will practice changing habits incrementally rather than all at once.

One practice that we will talk more about when we discuss lifestyle habits is the importance of not eating late at night. If it is usually your habit to eat a few hours before you go to bed, then the first step toward abstaining from late-night eating is to not eat after 8:00 p.m. You would try that for a week or two and then work your way down to eating no later than 7:00 p.m. After a week of that routine, you would then not eat after 6:00 p.m. Eventually, not eating late at night will become your habit. Later in this book, we'll explore more specific ways to tailor how and when to eat based on our different constitutions.

If you have a habit of working two hours later than everyone else in the office, then you can spend a week working only an hour and a half past everyone else, and so on. Regardless of the behavior, it is possible to use time as a way to develop your practice.

Sometimes it is difficult to determine which behaviors are and are not excessive because our needs change from one day to the next. This is the significance of finding our inner guru, as it is only by trying these practices and observing how we feel in response to them over time that we really and truly know what will help us to find balance. As you continue to experiment with removing excess from your lifestyle, please know that it is one of the most difficult goals to work toward and will require a lot of perseverance before you come to what really and truly works for you. I have full confidence, however, that once we are determined to change, each of us has what it takes to succeed.

The next thing I remembered after crashing on my bed that morning was the phone ringing later that day. Loudly.

build willpower in small quantities

We can strengthen our willpower by changing excessive behaviors in small increments only. This helps us create a new direction and lifestyle. The following exercise, based on a person who consumes three glasses of wine, soda, coffee, or too much water each day, is just one sample of how we can build our willpower.

1. For two weeks, when you're ready for another drink, fill your glass or cup two-thirds full. You are still having three servings, but the amount is equivalent to only two.

2. After two weeks, either have only two of these reduced amounts, or reduce each glass to half its original amount.

3. After another two weeks, drink only one cup or glass, and continue to do so.

If you tried to drink only one glass right at the beginning of trying this exercise, it is likely that you would feel deprived and would crave more beverages. By building up your willpower more gradually, however, you increase your ability to overcome such obstacles.

build willpower through small changes in time

When you sit down to eat, take a bite of food and put down your fork or spoon (or, if you're eating with your hands, place the food back on the plate). Finish chewing your food before you serve yourself another bite. Eat like this for one week.

After the first week, put down your utensil or food, and focus on your breathing for a few breaths before picking it up for another bite. Eat like this for one week.

After the second week, put down your utensil or food, see what you are thinking about, and observe your breathing for a moment before picking it up for another bite. Eat like this for one week and beyond.

"Good morning, Sunshine," Benjamin said. It was two in the afternoon.

"Whaaa-haa-huh?" This was a new language I was trying to avoid speaking.

"Are you glad you decided to stop drinking when you did?" Benjamin asked.

"I didn't decide to stop drinking," I replied. "Drinking decided to stop me."

"I go through that every day," he said. I thought I heard Jessie saying something in the background that sounded like *lightweight*.

I might have considered Benjamin the nicest guy in the world, but he was also a classic example of an alcoholic. I couldn't handle that kind of experience once, let alone on a daily basis. I didn't need any of the training I would eventually get in India to know that drinking like that—or any excess at all—was not something my body or mind could tolerate. I said my good-byes. Ron had recently taught me about some herbal remedies, and I headed to the kitchen to try them out in a soothing tea.

Although I did bump into Benjamin from time to time after that night, we never hung out together again.

fill in the blank

Building willpower as a way to abstain from excessive behaviors is the final practice featured in Part Two. As this is an important step in solidifying a foundation for your practice as a whole, spend at least a week building your willpower before moving on to the next chapter. This week is also a good opportunity to continue trying the exercises provided in chapters 1–4.

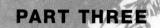

expression

posture practice and the pursuit of inner beauty

MY FIRST FEW WEEKS STUDYING at Arsha Yoga in India were intense but very satisfying. If I had thought that my initiation into this culture through a full schedule of classes, lectures, and ceremonies might settle into a more flexible routine, then I was greatly mistaken. The program outlined by my guru and the various other people administering the program created a schedule that allowed little time for leisure. Seeking outer pleasures was not emphasized on this path.

This suited me fine. I was here to learn. The Ayurveda classes were filled with relevant information, my guru's competent work with his patients assured me that I had made a good decision in coming here, and the simplicity of the environment they created provided me with a platform for investigating the tools I had sought in the first place.

The posture classes, however, were a bit of a surprise.

I had been studying and practicing yoga postures for some years, and like most people I knew in the West, I had been introduced to yoga through this physical practice. I was pleased with my progress through the system, for I was able to do things with my body that I hadn't been able to do earlier in my life. When I studied at ashrams, I found myself keeping up with the more advanced practitioners and could do most of the postures they did, and I had been one of the only people who could stand up on my forearms in the first level of teacher training. I was also proud of the fact that I was one of the only people I knew who had the discipline to practice postures at home on a fairly regular basis. However, I wasn't as open as many of the women, and I couldn't practice postures that required a great deal of flexibility, like full splits. This was okay, as there were many other ways to explore the practice.

The posture classes at Arsha were about an hour long. Much like the classes I had taken in the States, they started with gentle postures for warming up the body and then moved into more physically ambitious ones. My guru gave bits of information about the postures we were doing but said little else. The practice he offered seemed pretty tame compared to the more powerful sequences I had been taught in New York, and I had the sense that little emphasis was placed on this part of the practice.

About three weeks into my time there, the guru instructed the class to practice what I knew to be scorpion pose. It involved standing on one's forearms, much like I had done during my teacher training. However, the full expression of the posture involved raising the head and shoulders away from the floor, bending the knees so the feet lowered past the buttocks, and resting the feet on top of the head. I figured this was just the guru's way of teasing us, as I couldn't imagine someone actually doing such a thing in an environment so detached from practicing postures at all—let alone ridiculously hard ones.

I was wrong. When I emerged from my usual forearm stand, I looked up to see several of the people sustaining the full scorpion. Not only that, but their bodies weren't shaking, and they seemed to be putting no effort into the posture at all. For all I knew, they could have stayed like that for hours.

After class I approached two of the boys who had been practicing the scorpion. They, like many of those studying at the center, were teenagers who had been studying with this guru since they were young children.

"Can I ask you guys something?"

"Yes!" said Balu, the taller of the two boys. Shri, the shorter one, nodded with a smile.

"How did you do the scorpion so easily?" I asked.

Balu looked at Shri.

"What is a scorpion?" he said, turning back to me.

"Is it the name of one of those three cars in America?" Shri asked. Indeed, Shri was the one who had interrogated me about American music on my second day in India.

I laughed. "No, it's the posture you do when you're standing on your forearms and bringing your feet to your head."

"Oh, that," Balu said as he shrugged. "We do that to strengthen the spine."

"Well, sure," I said, "but it looked like it wasn't really any effort. People in the West spend hours a day trying to do that."

They looked at each other again. "Why do they spend hours a day? We don't really do it that much here."

"Well, you do practice more than that one class, right?"

"No," Balu said, "it's not really important."

I considered this for a moment. Then I thought of something else.

"Can you guys do full splits?"

Balu shrugged again. "Sure. Why not?"

It was then my turn to shrug. I really had no response. Why not indeed?

Over the time that I spent in India, we would have many more conversations like this. I would ask them about their posture practice, and they would reply something like "We don't think much about posture" or "We focus on meditation" or "Tell us more about the five cars!" I may have come to India very attached to how my posture practice had progressed and how my practice compared with that of other people. After a number of months, I started to let go of what my posture practice meant in relation to, well, pretty much anything except for how it opened my body for other practices.

My ultimate surprise, though, came even later. After I had stayed at the center for the second time, I stopped thinking about posture as much. My conversations with Shri and Balu even moved on to other, more important subjects, like what a hot dog was. I also lowered down to a full split for the very first time. Well, nearly.

the purpose of posture

Yoga postures are a series of physical poses that stretch, strengthen, and nurture the body. While this system is important to the practice that has been passed down over the centuries by my guru and other teachers, it is only one small part. Posture does have a role in the practice, but yoga includes much more. It does not place the same kind of emphasis on this physical aspect that we have placed on it in the West. In this chapter I intend not only to teach you how to practice certain postures for the sake of attaining balance, but also to show how the typical practicing of posture in the West is detrimental to this purpose.

Several thousand years ago, yoga was created by ancient sages in India as a system of training the mind to awaken to one's true self—the intended purpose of the practice outlined in this book. Yoga practice included many components, such as scholastic study, devotional chants, action for the betterment of all living things, and a variety of techniques based upon sitting in silence, such as controlled breathing and withdrawal of the senses. What these yogis found, though, was that there was a need to train the body to be capable of sustained periods of sitting. The body needed to be free of stiffness and pain, for if they were to sit all day in a cave somewhere in the mountains, they needed to be able to concentrate on their practice instead of on the pain in their knees or how much their lower backs hurt.

To develop a physical system, these sages began to observe how animals would wake from sleeping and then proceed to stretch themselves out before beginning the activities of their day. Given that these movements were performed by the animals out of a simple need to open their bodies and nothing else, the yogis considered them a natural and safe foundation for formalizing the opening of their own bodies. These movements eventually formed the basis of what we now know as postures.

With the use of this system, the yogis were able to stretch, strengthen, and nurture their bodies for their sitting sessions. They were able to lengthen and tone their muscles, purify their organs, and create greater overall health. Over the years, as yogis became more aware of the many physical and mental benefits of postures, the system expanded to include an ever-growing variety of ways to make the practice physical. When yoga became known in the West during the twentieth century, the system that had originally been intended as one component of the overall practice was received as a physical exercise and little else. Today, when most of us think of posture, we think of the fifty-person classes that are offered in yoga studios, the quick power session we can find in many gyms, and the tropical retreats available for practicing postures on the beach. These routines might include hints of the postures' original purpose, but focusing entirely on these kinds of experiences often causes greater imbalance in the form of injuries and other health problems. Later in this chapter I'll show you how an inappropriate posture practice can be detrimental to your balance.

The posture practice outlined in this chapter may surprise you in its intention and its execution. I intend for you to practice posture for the sake of opening your body and facilitating a greater sense of balance and ease in your everyday life. The people I observed in the class during my training in India may have been able to do particularly involved postures, but each one they practiced had a specific benefit and purpose. Their bodies naturally extended into them after many years of practice. You may know of people who practice certain systems of yoga posture, practice in certain spaces, wear certain types of yoga clothing, and go on pilgrimages to India to practice postures in certain environments, but I encourage you to use such tools only if it helps you on this path toward balance, happiness, and contentment.

discovering your beauty through posture

If we are to boil down the benefit of posture into its simplest form, then we can say that it opens the body. This is a worthwhile goal, for the more open the body, the more focused the mind. With a focused mind, we have a greater capacity to explore ways of finding contentment, peace, and all of the things that you promised yourself when you began the practices outlined in this book.

How can practicing a bunch of postures affect a person's mind? In Western forms of exercise, such as jogging, aerobics, and weight lifting, we work out to raise the heart level, burn fat, and attain what we think is a better body—or to maintain the better body we feel we already have. In contrast, the slower, more deliberate movement and organization of the body in posture practice requires investigating our limitations and committing ourselves to redefining those limitations. Because this investigation requires us to become more familiar with the difference between what we want ("I want to be flexible enough to come into a full split") and what we need ("I need to increase my flexibility so I increase cellular function"), we get to know ourselves from the inside out. Practicing in this way will help us to peel away inessential experiences and focus on beneficial actions. Working out for the sake of getting a better body is based on fears, such as thinking that if our bodies are not perfect, then we will not be accepted by others. When we turn our focus inward, we find exactly the body we're supposed to have. This, by itself, makes us beautiful—and will inspire us to gravitate toward similar, inwardly beautiful experiences.

With that said, there are many physical benefits to practicing posture. We often feel stiffness as a result of sitting at computers, driving in cars, walking long distances, breathing polluted air, eating too many unhealthy foods, relaxing in bed or on the sofa, and many other activities that are part of the modern world. This stiffness in the body is the evidence of poor circulation of energy, and stagnant energy leads to disease. When exercising and playing sports, one does not use every muscle in the body. Rather, a person overuses the same muscles and wears them out. In yoga posture, however, every part of the body is opened, and this stretching process stimulates blood flow, which in turn circulates oxygen. The increase of oxygen facilitates greater cellular function, which leads to a lower incidence of disease. Though this process is applicable on every level, a safe and purposeful practice of posture can help to resolve cardiovascular distress, improve circulation, improve glandular function, resolve acidity in the stomach, resolve issues of the nervous system, and many other benefits. Posture is intended to nurture—not tax—the mind and body.

In the West we work to tone our muscles and keep in shape. To maintain a healthy lifestyle it is certainly helpful to remain active, but excessively practicing the contractive movements of workout systems will shorten the muscles and place stress on the joints. With shorter muscles, less oxygen is finding its way to the cells, creating imbalance and stiffness in the body.

This imbalance can manifest in physical ways, such as inflammation, and emotional ways, such as anxiety and irritability. Consider how often our emotions manifest as physical conditions, such as the sensation of getting butterflies in the stomach when we're nervous or getting flushed in the face when we're embarrassed. This relationship between emotions and our bodies works in reverse as well: when we create tension and contraction in the body, it exists as tension and contraction in the mind and the organs, making them prematurely older.

The posture practice provided in the next section is intended to start you off down this path. If you find that you want to make posture a more abundant part of your practice, other resources will be made available to you. The chapters in this book are designed to complement one another in one cohesive practice, so be sure to know your intention as it relates to this general path before starting the physical components.

the twelve-posture sequence

According to some sources, there are over nine hundred different yoga postures available for practicing. Many books, posters, and other publications show different variations and sequences for pursuing this practice. With all of these postures and sequences available, forming your own practice can be an overwhelming task. In this section I am presenting you with a basic sequence of twelve postures that you can practice so that you can begin enjoying the benefits of this system right away.

These twelve postures have been chosen to provide you with a basic means of opening both the front and back of the body as well as improving circulation, aiding digestion, and nurturing the nervous system. Some postures are more active for warming up the body, and others are more passive for allowing the body to recover from the stresses of daily life. I recommend you begin practicing this sequence in the order it is provided, and as you grow more comfortable with it you can improvise as the guru in you deems appropriate. Please also keep the following points in mind when practicing this sequence.

The breath is as key to a good posture practice as it is to staying alive. The breath needs to be constant and never held. Once you follow the basic instructions provided for you in aligning yourself in the posture, forget about alignment and focus on breathing. This is the most important tool for opening up the body, as it will help you to release tension and increase your concentration—which is one of the practices to follow after posture.

Breathe in and out of your nose to retain energy and focus. Breathing out of your mouth can leave you feeling winded, as the air is forced out very quickly. Breathing through your nose can help you to remain present in your practice and can remind you to take deeper breaths. If the nose is blocked, then breathe through the mouth.

Our intentions are more important than the length of time we practice. Many of us define our exercise routines by the length of time we commit to them. Rather than determine your routine by how long you practice, notice how your body and mind feel at the beginning of the sequence. If you're feeling particularly stiff, take more time with each posture. If you're feeling light and open, consider taking less time with each posture but extend the muscles further to increase the stretch. As with everything in life, the greater the effort, the greater the benefit. Just remember, however, that sometimes the greatest effort is to let go of whether or not we've practiced long enough.

Practice each posture only one time per sequence. In the beginning, practice each posture for a couple of minutes as a general guideline. If you feel compelled to stay in certain postures for a greater length of time, then by all means explore that instinct. If a posture has a particularly good effect on you, such as a longer hold in child's pose helping to resolve stress, then stay in it longer. Once you've practiced regularly for months or even years, you can add more postures. This depends on your dedication.

Feel the stretch in the correct area. The instructions will say where on the body it is intended for you to be opening or feeling a stretch, so be sure to observe whether or not you are feeling the stretch in the correct area.

Mind the breath during the transitions between postures. These postures are arranged to aid your ability to go from one to the next while still focusing on your breathing. Breathing will help you to avoid injuries during transitions from one posture to another or coming in and out of postures, which is the most common time for injury to occur. There will therefore be times, especially at the beginning of your practice, that your body will need your careful guidance when transitioning from one posture to another. Your consistent and mindful breath will be your greatest and most important tool for ensuring the safety and deepening of your practice.

. . .

Visit yogicameron.com to view videos that will accompany the following postures.

posture 1: **downward-facing dog**

Press the arms into the floor.

Press the heels toward the floor.

Keep the hands and feet parallel to each other.

Breathe.

Many people associate yoga postures with downward-facing dog, and with good reason. Downward-facing dog is a useful posture with a variety of benefits and forms the foundation of many sequences. Practicing this posture stretches the major muscle groups of the entire back and back of the legs. We start the sequence with this posture because it helps us attain an openness and flexibility in the back of the torso and the front and back of the legs. This can help us enter into many other postures with greater ease.

How do I practice a safe downward-facing dog?

- Keep your weight distributed as evenly as possible in the arms and legs so as not to put too much pressure on the wrists or the spine.

- Keep the curvature of the spine as close to neutral as possible without overextending.

What are the benefits of downward-facing dog?

- It opens our back torso and the front and back of our legs.

- It builds strength in the arms and the rest of the upper body.

- It raises the pelvis above the heart (that is, an inversion), which in longer holds can lead to a relaxation of the organs.

posture 2: **low crescent lunge**

Bend the knee of the front leg in a right angle.

Bring the knee beyond the foot if you are more flexible.

Place the back leg in a straight line beyond the buttocks.

Allow the spine to be erect or bending backward.

Breathe.

Low crescent lunge is a useful posture for the beginning of a sequence for it opens up muscles in the groin area. This area needs to be open for deepening our practice into other postures, and especially for most sitting postures. From downward-facing dog, bring your right foot forward to begin the first half of low crescent lunge. The posture will need to be practiced on both sides for equal amounts of time.

How do I practice a safe low crescent lunge?

- Be sure to bend in the upper back when arching backward, and do not crunch in the lower back.

What are the benefits of low crescent lunge?

- It stretches the muscles in the groin region.

- It stretches the muscles in the lower back when arching backward.

- It serves as a warm-up for other postures.

posture 3: **cobra**

When on the floor, press into the hands as the chest comes forward and up.

Place weight in the arms to avoid crunching in the lower back.

Slightly bend the arms.

Allow the shoulders to relax down, and do not lift up by the ears.

Breathe.

Cobra is a posture intended to open up the muscles surrounding the spine. This will make the body more supple and elastic for breathing and sitting practices. As bending the spine backward is not a common way to move the body, it is important not to push into the posture but instead move into it gently. Move as far into the posture as feels right for your muscles at that particular moment. From low crescent lunge on the second side, return to downward-facing dog, place your knees on the floor, and lower the torso to the floor for cobra.

How do I practice a safe cobra?

- If you have been injured in the lower back region, be especially gentle when coming in and out of the posture, and be very sure to use the breath during these transitions.

What are the benefits of cobra?

- It stretches and tones the back muscles.

- It corrects displaced or damaged vertebrae over time.

- It aids digestion.

posture 4: **child's pose**

Place the arms pointing backward next to the body.

Allow the forehead to rest on the floor.

Breathe.

Child's pose allows us to emulate the experience in the mother's womb by curling up and being alone in a bundle. Instructors often teach their students to come back to this posture when they need to rest from the rigor of other postures, as it is very grounding and nurturing. Practicing child's pose can help us to release stress or emotions through easy breathing and rest. This posture follows cobra to allow for rest following the more active beginning of the sequence.

How do I practice a safe child's pose?

- Don't fall asleep!

What are the benefits of child's pose?

- It lowers the heart rate and blood pressure.

- It restores calmness to the entire system.

- It provides a stretch to the thighs and spine.

- It applies pressure to the abdomen and colon, which strengthens them.

- It helps resolve headaches and feelings of depression.

posture 5: **hero's pose**

Sit back on the heels.

Keep the spine erect.

Keep the hands on the knees.

Close the eyes.

Breathe.

If child's pose is a useful tool for restoring calm and grounding ourselves, then practicing hero's pose is a powerful opportunity to bring focus back to the breath. As hero's pose helps to bring focus to the breath and therefore the mind, it is a useful tool for exploring meditation.

What are the benefits of hero's pose?

- It helps to resolve issues of the knee.

- It stretches and opens the front thigh muscles.

- It helps to calm the nervous system when sat in for some time.

- It is great for resolving stress and anxiety.

posture 6: **legs-up-the-wall**

Rest the spine on the floor.

Rest the buttocks against the wall with the legs going up.

Rest the arms next to the torso.

Close the eyes and stay for three to five minutes.

Breathe.

The beginning of the sequence starts you off with downward-facing dog, which I suggested was an inversion. Legs-up-the-wall is another inversion, though it is a restful alternative to more demanding postures like headstand. Inversions allow the blood force to flow in the opposite direction from what it flows when we are upright, which increases blood flow—and therefore oxygen flow—to the head region. Find an unobstructed wall near where you're practicing to include this posture in your sequence, or just hold the legs up in the air.

What are the benefits of legs-up-the-wall?

- It rests the legs from fatigue.

- It reverses the intensity of blood flow, which helps resolve migraines, headaches, and other issues related to the head.

- It can relieve sinus congestion.

posture 7: **bridge (half wheel)**

Bring the feet close to the buttocks.

Interlace the fingers under the buttocks.

Lift the pelvis toward the sky.

To avoid tightening the buttocks,
press down the arms.

Breathe.

Bridge, along with other back bends like cobra, helps to develop health and flexibility in the spine. Having a healthy spine helps us to feel more comfortable during sitting and breathing practices. It also helps us to feel less nervous and more peaceful. While other, more aggressive back bends require much more flexibility in the spine and strength in the arms, bridge offers us a safe and simple way to explore this movement of the body.

How do I practice a safe bridge?

- Be sure to avoid applying pressure to the neck.

What are the benefits of bridge?

- It relaxes the nervous system while the spine is extended.

- It tones the thighs and shoulders.

posture practice and the pursuit of inner beauty

posture 8: **seated forward bend**

Place the legs parallel with the feet together.

Place the arms at the sides of the legs.

Draw the torso forward with a
little extended effort.

Keep the spine in its
natural alignment.

Breathe.

Like child's pose, the seated forward bend helps to nurture the body. While it can build serenity in the system, it may also bring deeply held emotions to the surface. Because of this, many people don't like staying in this posture for very long. Most who practice this posture are not able to bend very far forward until they've been practicing postures for some time. Be sure to stay focused on the breath as you turn yourself over during the transition from bridge.

How do I practice a safe seated forward bend?

- Avoid hunching over in the back.

- Avoid forcing the torso forward.

What are the benefits of seated forward bend?

- It increases flexibility in the legs and spine.

- It helps resolve heart and kidney issues.

- It aids digestion.

- It brings calmness and peace to the mind.

- It benefits those who are sad or angry.

posture 9: **spinal twist**

Sit up tall.

Hug the knee with the opposite arm.

The back arm assists with twisting.

Breathe.

The health of the spine is of the utmost importance when creating space in the body. Postures that rotate the spine, like the spinal twist, relax the central nervous system. As the nervous system governs the mental and physical health of our entire bodies, practicing this posture and others like it benefits the whole being. Be sure to practice the posture on both sides an equal amount of time.

How do I practice a safe spinal twist?

- Be sure not to place too much pressure on or lean back on the extended arm.

- If you have endured a spinal injury, be sure to be particularly gentle and pay greater attention to your breathing.

What are the benefits of the spinal twist?

- It relaxes the nerves and therefore the nervous system.

- It aids digestion.

- It helps the liver detoxify.

- It makes the back more flexible for better health.

posture 10: **butterfly**

While sitting, place heels evenly together.

Beginners: Place hands behind your body
for gentle lowering of legs.

When your legs are close to the floor, your
hands can gently press down on your legs.

Breathe.

As your posture sequence winds down, you can use butterfly to open the groin muscles for seated postures. Its placement toward the end will serve as preparation for the breathing and meditation exercises that are described in later chapters. Practicing butterfly centers on increasing the flexibility of the inner legs through a very gentle and gradual exploration. While many may like to flop down with a curved spine and touch the head to the floor in front of them, this offers little value to the practice until your legs are fully touching the ground and your back is flat.

How do I practice a safe butterfly?

- Be patient and gentle as you gradually open up the muscles.

- Don't force the legs down toward the ground.

- You can use the wall for support.

What are the benefits of butterfly?

- It builds elasticity of the inner thighs and groin area.

- It is stimulating to the pelvis and abdomen.

- When bending forward, it benefits the urinary bladder, kidneys, and health of the back.

posture 11: **corpse**

While lying down, widen the arms and feet to the point of letting go of the whole body.

Turn the palms facing upward.

Release any part of the body being held.

Breathe.

Many people's yoga practices end with a corpse posture, as it is the best posture for relaxing and surrendering the entire body to the ground. The arrangement of the body allows the earth to completely support us, and we can let go of our physical self. As such, corpse is for letting go of the ego and any fears we may be holding onto. Those who have difficulty letting themselves go may have a similar difficulty in trusting themselves.

How do I practice a safe corpse?

- In this practice, the body is asleep but the mind is awake and alert.

- Allow the mind to become fully aware of what the body is experiencing.

What are the benefits of corpse?

- Giving our bodies to the earth helps us to feel supported and grounded.

- It helps every organ of the body feel less tired and overworked.

- It helps the body distribute the energy that grows from the practice and the release of stress.

posture 12: **sitting pose**

Sit up tall with the legs crossed in front of the torso.

Relax and let the legs just be.

Sit on one or two cushions if having difficulty in the posture.

With cushions, a stretch should be felt in the groin area.

Breathe.

For the thousands of years that humanity existed before the use of modern chairs, people sat in this posture. Sitting in this way gives full support to the spine and nervous system and relieves the body of any stiffness experienced by sitting on sofas and chairs. While it may seem easy, it takes effort to sit in this way, and it is this effort that develops a person's willpower. The sitting pose is featured at the end of this sequence as a segue into a breathing and meditation practice and as an opportunity to begin incorporating it into your daily life.

How do I practice a safe sitting pose?

- Be sure to remain focused, or you may start to levitate! (Smile. It may happen.)

What are the benefits of the sitting pose?

- It allows the mind to stay alert.

- When practiced correctly, there is no stiffness and circulation is perfect.

creating a practice with postures

Beverly was a client who had tried practicing yoga postures but had developed an injury. While practicing an aggressive form of power yoga taught to her by a private instructor, she forced herself into a certain posture and injured her lower back. Her whole body locked up as a result, and she couldn't even move without experiencing pain. Beverly worked as a preschool teacher, and because this back injury lasted for several months, she spent that time barely making it through the workday, let alone being able to run around with her students and participate in the active games that preschoolers enjoy.

As Beverly was a person who liked to be on the go and had always incorporated some form of exercise into her life, she was eager to return to high-impact physical activity once she recovered from her injury. When I met her, she had been jogging and lifting weights an hour and a half a day for about six months. However, she told me during the consultation at the beginning of our first session that she tended to feel sore and even drained as she finished up her workouts.

Beverly and I worked together over the course of several weeks. At first she feared another back injury and was apprehensive about trying postures again, but when I introduced her to the slow, meditative sequence I found to be appropriate to counteract her particularly active lifestyle, she was open to trying it. We discussed how she was feeling at the beginning of each session and whether or not she had encountered any obstacles related or unrelated to her practice. As the sessions progressed, her body started to open up more and more, and she seemed to be letting go of her need for constant activity.

One morning, about halfway through her practice, I decided to introduce her to a certain posture that would help her regulate some of her hormonal activity, and doing this pose required her to lie on her back and bring her legs over her head. Because she had been warmed up by the first half of the practice, I was very surprised to observe her whole body seize up when she entered this posture. She held her breath for moments at a time. Every movement hurt. She made a comment about being down for the count again, convinced she was once again going to be out of commission for several months and unable to do her job. Tears started to roll down her face. I worked with her on her breathing, got her to extend her legs while she was on her back, took her through a series of gentle postures, and massaged the area on her lower back that was the focal point of her pain. Within fifteen to twenty minutes, she was moving around on the floor with very little pain, and after thirty minutes she was walking with nothing more than a little soreness.

Beverly had left a crucial piece of information out of our chat at the beginning of the morning. Earlier that day she had gotten very upset with someone and had a verbal confrontation. She brought that stress and tension into the session. Had news of this incident been included in our chat, I would not have recommended that she practice the particular posture that had triggered the old injury. When her body locked up, she began to hold onto the fear that she would not be able to move around in her job and in other parts of her life. This, in turn, caused her to create even more tension in her body.

While it might seem that the yoga posture was responsible for Beverly reinjuring herself, the injury was simply lying dormant from many months earlier. The tension left over from her confrontation earlier in the day made her more vulnerable to the weakness in her back. It's likely that had she been exerting herself with weights and running as per her old routine, she not only would have injured herself but might have done even greater damage than what happened with the yoga postures. Much of back pain and injury centers on the dysfunction of the nervous system, so it was no surprise that Beverly's injury was related to a problematic nerve. The only way for her to work through such a problem was to breathe through it, as doing so would help her to release her fears surrounding the injury and alleviate the pain in her back.

This is a particularly important story for me to share with you for several reasons. First, it shows how an appropriate use of yoga posture can be a very effective tool for uncovering the problems and imbalances we hold in our bodies as a result of the stress of day-to-day life. Postures can help us to work through injury, as was the case when the routine I conducted with Beverly helped her to breathe into her pain and strengthen the nervous system to the point of successfully alleviating the back complaints. When we increase the blood flow to the muscles and tendons surrounding the central nervous system in the back and succeed in calming the mind, we both relieve tension in the back and send healthier messages to the brain. This release of tension in the nervous system leads to a relief of back pain.

The story also shows that our emotions and thoughts have a very real impact on our bodies, as Beverly's confrontation took place at a separate time from her experience with the problematic yoga posture, and yet she still experienced physical ramifications hours later. What is most important, however, is that Beverly's go-go-go approach to her physical well-being through power yoga and then high-impact exercise was not a proper match for her go-go-go lifestyle in her job and the rest of her life.

A POSTURE PRACTICE IS UNIQUE TO THE PERSON

Creating a practice through postures is a very individual process. While there are certain postures that are recommended for most—if not all—people, the frequency, intensity, and composition of the practice will vary from person to person. Practicing postures is very important in the early part of the process of finding the guru in you. When you teach yourself which postures are or are not appropriate for your immediate needs, you will better understand how to relate to the present moment. It is in the present moment that you will cultivate a greater understanding of yourself.

People like Beverly are always on the move, and therefore they are typically drawn to faster yoga and other aggressive physical disciplines that mirror their mentality. Other people who are more slow-paced and laid-back tend to crave a low-impact type of activity—if they engage in a physical activity at all. When your posture practice mirrors your imbalances (I feel lethargic, therefore I'm not going to practice posture; I feel stressed, therefore I'm going to push myself harder; I feel scattered, therefore I'm not going to focus too much on any one posture), it only furthers those imbalances and has a negative impact on your health. At the beginning of the chapter I suggested that the way people in the West relate to posture can be to our detriment, and in saying that I was alluding to how likely we are to use this system to perpetuate our fears instead of challenging ourselves to observe exactly what we need for our bodies to be open and healthy.

You are the best judge of whether your posture practice should be more active in response to a slower-paced lifestyle, more relaxing in response to an always-on-the-go lifestyle, or a combination of more than one factor. Below are guidelines for people with different needs to follow when practicing the posture sequence outlined above or some other system. Additionally, the later chapter on Ayurveda will provide a different set of guidelines for how to approach posture based on assessing your body's constitution.

I've never practiced yoga postures before: Try practicing the sequence of twelve postures in this chapter, spending several minutes in each pose. The practice as a whole will probably take between twenty and thirty minutes.

I'm always on the move and do high-impact cardiovascular and weight training: Try practicing the sequence in this chapter with a particular emphasis on child's pose, hero's pose, legs-up-the-wall, and corpse. These more calming postures should account for at least half of your practice. Also consider taking a restorative yoga class under an experienced teacher's direction.

I'd like to try practicing these postures, but I feel so tired and lethargic all the time that it seems easier to skip it. Try practicing the more active postures, like downward-facing dog, cobra, spinal twist, and low crescent lunge for longer periods of time, or repeat them in a short sequence before moving on to the remainder of the twelve poses. This will increase blood flow, which will increase oxygen to the brain and spark a greater need for activity. Consider also trying a beginner-level Vinyasa or Ashtanga yoga class under the supervision of an experienced teacher.

I haven't worked out in years, I'm overweight, and I can't really move much at all: Begin practicing the simplest postures like hero's pose, child's pose, legs-up-the-wall, and corpse pose for a few minutes each. These postures should feel relaxing, but if you feel any discomfort then come out of the posture and take a few deep breaths before trying again.

The only time of day I can create a practice for myself is late at night. Whenever I exercise at night, I can't sleep: Practice the simple postures like hero's pose, child's pose, legs-up-the-wall, and corpse. This is better than not practicing any postures at all, for while they will be a source of calm and relaxation, they will also be an opportunity for you to work with the breath.

As you continue to explore posture as a part of your practice, you'll find that there are many different methods, systems, and even brands requiring certain routines and commitments for the sake of practicing. Many students I've worked with have commented that yoga posture sequences in studios and gyms seem to be complicated and even forced. If I communicate nothing else in this chapter, I hope to make it clear that the practice of posture is not the end goal of the path of yoga, and it is not supposed to be as difficult as it often appears in the Western yoga industry. Posture is a wonderful tool for stripping away inessential aspects of your life, but I hope you commit as much energy to letting go of it as to practicing it.

. . .

I returned to India last year to study for several weeks under my guru, as I do every year. On my way to India, sitting in a hard plastic chair on a long layover in London, I reflected on an interesting pattern. When living in the United States, I'm not quite as open in my body as I am when I return to Arsha Yoga. At the ashram there are no phone calls, no text messages (and little computer use), no sofas, and no Western foods or restaurants. The simplicity of this lifestyle along with the total immersion in yoga and Ayurveda are what I find so appealing about training there. After a few weeks of this lifestyle I am always able to lower my hips to the ground in a full split. Thanks to text messages and hard plastic seats, though, in the West my hips are about as far from the floor as I am from India. Well, nearly.

I laughed to myself. Though it had not been an effortless transition, I was pleased to note how little splits and scorpions mattered anymore. That day I had practiced posture for only forty-five minutes, and yet my body felt strong and my mind alert.

I may have been sitting on a hard seat in an airport waiting for a delayed plane, but still I was happy.

After all, this is the true purpose of yoga.

fill in the blank

As you will learn in later chapters, posture is traditionally followed by other daily practices based in the tradition of yoga. Incorporate the twelve-posture sequence into your morning schedule for at least a few days before reading chapter 7. This will serve as a first basic step in creating a daily routine of practice.

the breath

7

"THIS . . ."
Thwack.
"is . . ."
Thwack.
"absolutely . . ."
Thwack.
"unacceptable!"
Thwack.

The man banged his suitcase handle on the counter with each word he yelled at the airline employee. His wife stood behind and to the side of him, holding their daughter. The daughter couldn't have been older than one.

"Sir," said the employee, "I understand that this has been an inconvenience to you, and on behalf of the airline I apologize—"

"An inconvenience? *An inconvenience?*" he roared. "You're goddamned right it's an inconvenience! My suitcase is ruined, and it's *your airline's fault!*"

"Sir—"

"When I checked my suitcase in, it was whole, and now it's in pieces!"

"Sir, please—"

"*You* broke it!"

"Honey—" said his wife.

"No! They broke our suitcase handle! I want this fixed!" *Thwack.* "I want somebody's ass—" *thwack* "—right—" *thwack* "—now!"

Listening to a verbal assault on an airline employee didn't seem like a particularly productive way to be spending my morning, but I didn't see any other choice. The day before, I had flown to Los Angeles to work with a client for the week. Upon my arrival I had discovered that my bag with clothes and toiletries showed up just fine on the luggage carousel, but my bag filled with the herbs, oils, and other treatment tools I was to use with my client did not. This particular client had an overactive lifestyle and certain health issues for which I needed the calming influence of the oils and herbs. It seemed necessary to have everything available for our work together, particularly because she had been putting off the appointment for some months and I had traveled three thousand miles to conduct these treatments.

"We're so sorry, sir," the man at the baggage claim office had said to me the day before when I realized my bag wasn't coming off the conveyer belt. "It looks like that particular bag didn't make the trip to LA on that same flight from New York."

"Does that mean the bag is lost?" I asked. It held several thousand dollars' worth of materials and tools.

"Oh, no, of course not. It will simply have to come on a later flight."

"A later flight," I repeated. "When can I pick it up?"

He checked his computer. I hoped I wouldn't have to stay at the airport for more than an hour or two, as my client was expecting me that evening. She lived about ten miles from LAX, which in LA traffic would take about an hour and a half. If I got there early enough, I'd be able to start her on an early bedtime routine right away.

"It should be here by tomorrow morning."

"Tomorrow—morning?" I blinked.

"Oh, yes," he said, sounding rather pleased. "It would usually take several days, but we've made it a priority to get missing bags from this flight here right away."

I considered this for a moment.

"Right," I said. "Thank—thank you for your time."

So I had begun the work with my client that evening, but the herbal treatments were put on hold. While we did get that early bedtime routine started right away, we needed to focus on other practices like posture until I worked out the situation with my luggage. It would be fine.

I returned to LAX the next morning to claim my bag, where I found myself in line behind the man shouting at the airline employee.

"Get me a manager!" *Thwack.* "Get me a muther-effin' supervisor, *now!*"

This man not only was holding up the line because of a suitcase handle, but his pounding of the handle suggested that he could very well become a physical threat. As his tantrum was keeping me from claiming my bag, I was forced to stand there and watch his agitation grow. I wondered what I might do if things got even worse. *Take the man down,* said a small voice. *But your karate is horrible,* said a different, louder voice. Given that I was there to claim materials that would help someone foster a greater sense of calm in her life, the fact that I had come across a less-than-calm situation was a great yogic irony. If I wanted that bag, I had to endure his hostility toward an undeserving woman. Given the tension of the situation, however, it was significant that I was not actually experiencing any tension myself.

How was this possible? Wasn't this man being a complete ass? Didn't he deserve to be decked? Many people would not only have taken him down but also considered themselves heroes for doing so.

My lack of tension did not come from my having a stronger moral center or being a superior being.

It came from the breath.

When he began slamming his handle on the counter, I closed my eyes and began to inhale through my nose. I allowed my abdomen to expand, and then my lungs followed suit. I inhaled for several counts and then exhaled through my nose for twice as long. I repeated this several times before I opened my eyes.

Eventually he stopped slamming the handle on the counter, and I noted three things: (1) This man, while less agitated, was not about to leave anytime soon. (2) He posed no threat to the woman, outside of her likely getting a headache by the end of the exchange. (3) Rather than feel annoyed and disturbed by this man and the barrier he had placed between me and my missing bag, I was simply watching him as if he were on a movie screen.

It was possible that I would find my bag somewhere in the baggage claim area without the help and guidance of the airline employee, and it was possible I wouldn't. She had enough to deal with for the moment, so I not only let go of my disapproval of this situation, I also let go of whatever happened to my possessions as well. I left the office and sought out the baggage claim carousels.

breathing without a windshield or headlights

A lot of things happened in the above story. An airline delayed the arrival of my bag. A man yelled at another human being. I observed but didn't participate in the tension of the room. I let go of the bag and the situation that was keeping me from finding it. I gave up control. The story relates in several ways to the practice outlined in this book, from the violence this man was exhibiting toward the airline employee to the attachment I felt to getting my bag to the detachment I found on the second day. I share this experience with you, though, not because of the behaviors of the various people in the story, but because I was able to attain a sense of balance through the use of my breath. For this step of the practice, we learn to become aware of the breath and to use it in all circumstances. This is known as conscious breathing.

Breathing is necessary for sustaining human life. Each one of us requires oxygen to live, and the process of inhaling oxygen and then exhaling carbon dioxide is a vital part of ensuring proper functioning of the body's many physiological systems. Many of us, however, take breathing for granted. It becomes an unconscious act that may sustain us but does not necessarily enrich us. We often take quick, shallow breaths or even hold our breath outright without even realizing it. Yogic tradition teaches us that this stifled form of breathing is a major contributing factor to the suffering we endure in our everyday lives.

Consider what would happen if you drove a car that had four wheels, an engine, an undercarriage, a steering wheel, brakes, and a seat for the driver—but nothing else. It didn't have a body, it didn't have other seats, it didn't have headlights, it didn't have turn signals, it didn't have a windshield, and it didn't have a speedometer. What would driving this car be like? The car would get you from point A to point B, but it would do so with the wind and rain overwhelming you from every direction, you wouldn't know if you were traveling at a safe speed, you wouldn't be able to see anything in the dark, and other drivers wouldn't know when you were turning or changing lanes. If passengers rode with you in (or, technically, on) the car, they would be sprawled out over the uncomfortable metal bed of the undercarriage and would be in serious danger of falling off. It sounds absurd, doesn't it? The act of taking shallow or no breaths in our day-to-day lives is like driving a car without these many parts: it might help us to remain alive, but the quality of that life is poor and vulnerable to an awful lot of rainy days.

Earlier we explored how succumbing to the senses can lead us to feel attached to objects, relationships, or other aspects of our lives. Then we explored how those attachments lead to an indulging of the senses through excessive behaviors. Present throughout all of these behaviors, however, is the breath. If we live a life without conscious breathing, we are allowing the breath to fall into rhythm with whatever our senses are picking up around us. We hold our breath out of fear when watching a scary movie. We begin panting after rich foods we see in the display case of a bakery. When we allow our emotions to prompt shallow and short breaths, we are much more likely to indulge in the fears and disturbances that lead to excessive and even destructive behaviors. We allow our senses to drag us around.

To bring awareness to our breathing is to bring balance to our lives. This begins with the practice of controlling the breath.

conscious breathing

The act of conscious breathing is one of the fundamental practices of yoga. This practice can manifest through a variety of different exercises and techniques, but the overall intention is to control the emotional reactions we experience as a product of our senses and by doing so to control the mind. When we control the mind through the breath, we become masters of our own bodies. You may have noticed, in the previous chapter on practicing postures, how consistently I reminded you to breathe. The stretching and strengthening movements of the postures may seem like the primary ingredient in opening the body, but it is in fact the use of the breath in relation to those movements that creates the suppleness. Many yogis who have committed to the practice of controlling their breathing have become so masterful over the functions of their bodies that they can spend periods of time not even breathing at all.

It is not the intention of this chapter to provide an anatomy lesson on the relationship of the lungs to the rest of the body. However, it is helpful to explore certain aspects of this process to understand why bringing consciousness to the breath is so central to attaining a life of peace and joy. When we breathe, we take in oxygen, which is crucially important to cellular function. From our lungs, our blood then delivers this oxygen to our entire bodies. When we take quick, shallow breaths, we are using only a small portion of our lungs' overall capacity, and this more erratic use of the respiratory system makes it less efficient at delivering oxygen to our bodies. With less efficient oxygen intake, our cellular function decreases to the point that disease and other imbalances emerge throughout the body. The flip side of this problem, of course, is the use of the breath as a tool: when we increase the efficiency of our breathing, we not only reduce the occurrence of disease and imbalance, but we also create greater prosperity in all of our biological functions and thought patterns.

Human beings take on average from twelve to twenty breaths per minute. In the yoga world it is popular to illustrate the relationship of breath efficiency to longevity by referring to Paramahansa Yogananda's discussion of animals who live a long time. Yogananda is known throughout the West for his influential book *Autobiography of a Yogi,* and entire communities have been organized around his teachings. He shows that animals that live longer tend to take fewer breaths per minute, the most noted example of this being the giant tortoise, which can live to be well over one hundred fifty years old—and yet it breathes only four times per minute. Other animals that live longer include the elephant, which breathes an average of four to five times per minute, and horses, which breathe as little as eight times per minute. In contrast, animals that take a greater number of breaths per minute live a much shorter period of time. These animals include the chipmunk, which breathes ninety-five times per minute, and the mouse, which breathes one hundred sixty times per minute.

As we use more of our lung capacity and take fewer breaths, we build the body's ability to function in the way that has been intended for us by nature. Unlike the many animals cited by people like Yogananda, however, we have the option to control the breath through specific exercises and thus increase our potential for living longer and healthier lives.

marie

Marie was a television producer who said, when she contacted me, that she was frustrated with her fast-paced lifestyle. She told me that she never felt that she had time for anything, even though she was getting things done all the time. She often found herself unable to sit still for more than a few minutes.

When I arrived at her home, I found that Marie's gaze traveled all over the room, rarely focusing on any one thing. In addition, our discussion of the work we would do together that week was interrupted by a rather loud pounding noise coming from right outside her home— construction with

the guru in you

jackhammers and other devices. Marie became distracted, and although we tried to continue our conversation, her eyes and even limbs started to go haywire.

After apologizing to me, she got up and went outside. A minute later she returned, saying she had asked the man with the jackhammer to stop and he would take a break. We continued to talk, but five minutes later the noise was back. Marie looked restless, and her face started to show signs of anger and resentment. She glanced at the door, and I guessed she was ready to go out again and yell at the crew.

I asked her to close her eyes. She looked at me for a moment and then did so. I pointed out to her that, while this noise was very loud and present to the space we were sharing in that moment, it was simply an alarm. "It's definitely alarming," she responded. I clarified that what I meant was that this noise, like every other noise we hear during our practice and through-out our lives, can be used as an alarm clock that notifies us that we need to return to the breath. "When the sound occurs," I said to her, "we come back to the breath instead of getting involved with the sound itself." I had her breathe in through her nostrils so that her stomach then her lungs expanded, and then breathe out all of the air through her nostrils for twice the length of time of the inhalation. She repeated this several times.

We resumed our conversation without my asking her how she felt, as I didn't want her thinking about the noise at all. Even though the jack-hammer continued on, we were able to talk. I learned that she had taken a number of yoga classes before, and it wasn't surprising to learn that she liked the aggressive heated yoga classes. When I asked whether she had practiced breathing, she told me that she had practiced several breath-ing exercises, including alternate nostril breathing (described below) and advanced breathing exercises that build fire in the body.

I sat there for a moment and looked into her face. I was pleased to see that she held my gaze and was sitting quietly, without moving around. I then asked her to do the exercise we had just done as her entire breathing practice. She shifted in her seat and even questioned whether it would be enough to practice only that one exercise. In response, I told her sev-eral things: that for the first five years of my practice, I practiced only that exercise and the alternate nostril breathing she had mentioned; that while there was value in all those other practices, they were beneficial only in specific circumstances and doing some of them would even throw her out of balance; that they needed to be practiced only after many years of exploring other, more preliminary practices; and that even learned yogis who have conquered the mind have done so by the most simple of practices. Since she tended to be in constant motion, exercises that created more heat in the body would exacerbate the feeling that she was overwhelmed by her life.

For the rest of our week together, we continued to focus on that one exercise. By the end of that week, she had a great sense of focus and calm in both the practices we did together and the other tasks I saw her complete.

The jackhammers visited her for as long as I was there, though they never really bothered her again.

creating a practice with the breath

The above story, like my story at the airport, suggests how significant a role conscious breathing can play in developing our practice in our everyday lives. Marie not only used a simple exercise to draw her focus into the breath, but she also learned how beneficial a simple breathing practice can be.

In the previous chapter on postures, I provided a sequence of poses that ended with a sitting posture. I suggested that the sitting posture end the sequence because breathing exercises are the next step after postures and such exercises are often practiced in a basic, grounded seat. The remainder of this chapter is focused on exploring different ways we can use conscious breathing as a practice. It will show how we can incorporate the breath into our daily lives, as in Marie's and my stories, as well as how we use the breath after we've practiced postures.

A BREATHING PRACTICE IN OUR EVERYDAY LIVES

If we were to completely integrate conscious breathing into our lives, we would be emulating the breathing patterns of the elephants or giant tortoises and breathing only a few times per minute. We would be using our entire lung capacity for each breath, and this habit would remain constant for every moment that we're awake (with the exception of while we're doing different breathing exercises on our yoga mats).

This scenario will, of course, seem daunting for many of us. Such a supremely regulated breath may help us to balance our emotions and allow

the full breath

The full-breath exercise is a basic technique that requires us to use our entire lung capacity. In yoga communities, the name of this exercise is typically translated as "deep breath," but it seems deep only in comparison to the shallow breathing we're all used to. The intention of this exercise is to train ourselves to use our lungs fully to take in air and the life-giving oxygen that air provides.

The full breath is very simple. The first step is to inhale through the nose so that the abdomen begins to expand. About halfway through your inhale, you should notice your chest expanding as well, and even a tiny lifting of the shoulders. Please note, though, that by *expand,* I don't mean that you stick out your gut or force out your chest. Instead, your intake of air is substantial enough for there to be a natural expansion of these various parts of the body.

Next, exhale the air out of your lungs through the nose. First the chest relaxes, then the stomach is sucked in slightly to release all the air. There should be no holding of the breath anywhere in the inhale-exhale-inhale cycle. As you might remember from the above story about Marie, I had her inhale for a certain length of time and then spend twice that amount of time exhaling. This greater time for exhaling requires us to completely let go of the air in our lungs with control, which in turn heightens the respiratory system's efficiency.

You may remember this pattern of breathing from the earlier exercise called Sit Before You Veg. This is essentially the same practice, and I present it here in a chapter on breath not only to reiterate the importance of developing a conscious breathing practice, but also to demonstrate in how many different situations this basic practice can be used.

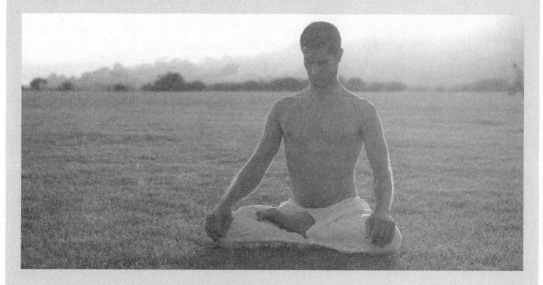

for a longer and prosperous life, but given how often we get distracted in any given moment, it doesn't seem like a realistic prospect. This is why it helps to start small and build this part of our breathing practice in specific parts of our lives. First, however, we must learn the full-breath exercise, which you've now seen not once but twice, in both Marie's and my stories. The exercise is described on page 143.

To incorporate conscious breathing into our everyday lives, we can use the full breath in specific situations and in specific ways. What follows is a list of situations through which the full breath can be used to overcome obstacles and begin forming a more consistent practice of conscious breathing throughout the day.

- *When presented with conflict:* At an airport or a grocery store or at work, we can find ourselves in a situation fraught with conflict and tension. Practice full breaths when you find yourself becoming tense in response to other people's behavior. Be conscious of this breathing until the tension has subsided.

- *When distracted by our environment:* Marie didn't think she could concentrate on our conversation when jackhammers were being used outside her house, but the full breath brought her back to the present moment. Whenever a noise or other distraction presents itself to you, use it like an alarm clock that notifies you to become aware of the breath.

- *When eating:* As the full breath is to be practiced through the nose, it is possible to practice and chew at the same time. Experiment with practicing the full breath each time you eat. This will require you to pay more attention to your eating and likely cause you to take more time to chew. It is the best weight-loss plan you'll ever find.

- *When waiting in line:* Many of us have felt frustrated while standing in a long line, be it at the post office, at the supermarket, or when waiting to buy movie tickets. Practicing full breath while in line not only will help you to develop greater patience, it will also give you something to focus on instead of the person in front of you who insists on paying for groceries in pennies.

- *When receiving bad news:* Many of us often hold our breath in an effort to brace ourselves for bad news. Breathing through the bad news gives us an opportunity to ease the tension that usually surrounds such an experience.

- *While talking:* This is one of the more complicated practices included. However, it is also one of the more important ones as the breath is constantly interrupted during conversations. If we are not conscious of our breath while having an emotionally heightened conversation with someone, we will find our breath cutting out and becoming erratic. If we talk late at night when we should be sleeping, or if we endure five- or six-hour meetings of continual talking, then we undermine our ability to breathe in a beneficial way. Being exposed to such detrimental routines on a regular basis will further increase our anxiety and can lead to migraines and other health issues.

Beyond everyday situations in our day-to-day lives, the full breath can also be incorporated into our formal breathing practice while on the yoga mat. The following section will teach you about developing your breathing practice as a continuation of the work you are doing with postures.

BEGINNING A SEATED BREATHING PRACTICE

As noted above, a component of our breathing practice is cultivated in a more formal way while in a seated posture. The postures we explored in the previous chapter were originally designed to create ease and openness in the body. When we open our bodies, we're then able to sit for extensive periods of time without pain. This idea of extensive sitting, of course, is not necessarily the goal of everyone who begins this type of practice, but breathing exercises like the ones described in this chapter can help us to calm the mind, develop concentration, and, as suggested throughout this chapter, improve our health and longevity.

Practicing postures like the twelve-posture sequence I provided in the previous chapter will help you to open up your body so that sitting while breathing is possible. When you come to the sitting posture at the end of the sequence, consider starting off with a basic breathing practice to supplement these other components of the practice you're developing.

Some of the techniques developed by the ancient yogis build heat, and others cool the body down. Some cultivate a greater abundance of life force while others have more of a cleansing effect on the system. As I suggested

alternate nostril breathing

According to the ancient yogis, when we allow our breathing to occur subconsciously, we inhale through one nostril for several hours and then inhale through the other nostril for several hours. This cycle continuously repeats throughout the day. When we are in optimal health, this transition from one nostril to the other happens every two hours. Since most of us are weighed down by the imbalances that occur in everyday life, this transition will often be out of balance and favor one nostril over the other for longer than two hours.

We've all heard of the idea that we have two sides of the brain. According to modern science, the left side controls our logical and reasoning abilities and the right side controls our creative activity. When we allow our breathing to be dominated by one nostril over the other, we create an imbalance in the brain activity of these complementary sides and

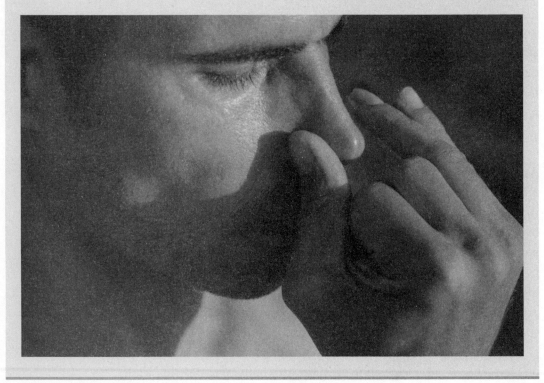

undermine the body's ability to maintain balance. According to yogic science, the body is in constant motion between opposing forces like hot and cold or active and passive, and alternate nostril breathing helps us to restore balance to the balance of male and female energies and calm the nervous system. This will help us to be open in both nostrils and, as the nose is the passage to the brain, we will enjoy a more balanced sense of awareness.

From your seated position, bring your left hand down to your left knee and lightly bring your thumb and forefinger together. With your right hand, touch your pointer finger and middle finger to the heel of your palm and bring your thumb and ring finger to either side of your nose. Close your eyes.

1. Gently press your right nostril closed with your thumb and exhale through your left nostril. Please note that during this practice we also continue the technique of full breath.

2. Inhale through the left nostril.

3. Block the left nostril with your ring finger and exhale through the right nostril.

4. Inhale through the right nostril.

5. Block the right nostril and continue the cycle.

If you forget where you are in the cycle, remember that the cycle consists of exhaling, inhaling, then blocking, then again exhaling, inhaling, then blocking, and continuing the cycle. Do not hold your breath at any point in the cycle, as it is not useful to work with breath retention until you are under the guidance of an experienced teacher and after many years of practice. Also, you may find that one or both nostrils feel blocked on any given day. If this is the case, and practicing the exercise requires you to force and push the air in and out, then forego the exercise for the day.

Alternate nostril breathing is a safe breathing practice to pursue, and the above steps can be repeated for as long as you feel balanced but have not strained yourself. Thirty minutes may be too little, and five minutes may be too long. You might remember Susan in chapter 4, who learned to use certain breathing techniques to restore balance to her body. As one of her primary issues was her attachment to her abusive boyfriend, I suggested alternate nostril breathing as a way to balance the male and female energies. In the next chapter we'll explore how to use specific components of alternate nostril breathing to resolve different types of energy imbalances in our bodies.

to Marie in the above story, while there may be many different techniques for us to choose from, practicing some of them in excess can create more imbalance than balance in the body and mind. You may also recall that I told Marie that I only used two breathing exercises for the first five years of my practice: the full breath and alternate nostril breathing. These basic techniques were taught to me by my guru and other teachers to form the foundation of my breathing practice, and I encourage you to spend some time practicing these techniques until you become more experienced with controlling the breath. The more complicated breathing practices should be taught to you at the correct moment and by a learned guide who has mastered the breath. They are few.

Using the full breath as part of a seated breathing practice is simple as well. When in the seated posture, rest both hands on the knees and lightly bring the thumb and index finger together. Straighten the arms so that they become a source of support in keeping the spine erect. Close the eyes. Inhale until the abdomen and chest expand, and then exhale until the chest deflates and the stomach is pulled in. Avoid forcing the air in and out, and instead allow the inhalation to be deep and the exhalation to be long and controlled. Over time, the exhalation will become twice as long as the inhalation. Repeat this cycle.

How long is an appropriate time for practicing one or both of the techniques? Our minds are typically influenced by numbers in everything that we do in our society. Rather than give you a fixed time limit, I would like you to start becoming aware of how long you should practice. Instead of setting an external clock, you will choose your practice time with your internal self, as you feel and become conscious of how much time is enough and how much is too little. If you tend to be an achiever, go gently. If you are a mover, be steady. If you are a sleeper, be more active. Let the guru in you be your guide.

There are a variety of ways to pursue conscious breathing in our lives, and more important than practicing for specific lengths of time or growing the ability to do exceptional things with our bodies is the simple act of committing ourselves to an awareness of the breath whenever we can. As with all aspects of this practice, it can start small in the beginning and grow as we move through different stages of our lives. While our time on this earth may offer us many obstacles and challenges as we drive from point A to point B, we at least have one thing that will remain constant throughout: we will always have our breath.

. . .

My quest to find my delayed bag had the exact ending one would expect. In the baggage claim area, two different carousels had luggage on them. The nearest one was active, and it was surrounded by people who had just arrived on an incoming flight. I decided to check the static carousel before lining up with everyone else at the moving one. No bag.

I joined the group at the moving carousel, squeezing in at the very end. A bright pink suitcase moved past, returning through the small doorway to the loading area. When the pink suitcase came around again, I knew that the carousel had completed a cycle. It completed a second cycle. And a third. Still, I remembered my full-breath exercise and committed myself only to watching each suitcase as it passed.

Halfway through the fourth cycle, I saw my bag. It must have been unloaded just as I was waiting. I was not surprised that I found it or that I had encountered obstacles before retrieving it. Life always offers us this type of challenge. In the end, I simply created an opportunity to breathe through it for the sake of growth.

fill in the blank

Having a breathing practice encourages a greater sense of mindfulness and awareness, which in turn helps us to be consistent in pursuing our sacred sense of self. Before expanding beyond the yogic practices outlined in this and previous chapters with the program outlined in chapter 8, spend at least several days practicing your breathing as a follow-up to your posture practice.

8

living the ayurveda way

three stories of three women

MARJORIE WELCOMED ME into her apartment. She appeared to be rather successful in her work as a film producer, as her space was large and abundant with light. The air conditioner was running full blast, even though it was only sixty-five degrees out on this sunny, dry desert day in Los Angeles.

"Can I offer you a drink?" Marjorie asked.

"No, thank you," I said. "I'm fine."

"You're sure?" she said. "It's really no trouble. I'm getting myself some water."

"Thank you, but I'm all set."

She went into the kitchen.

"Can I get you something to eat, or anything?" she called out through the doorway.

"No, really, I'm fine."

A minute or so later she returned with a large tumbler filled with ice and water. I noticed she was sweating a little.

"Did I do a good enough job with that questionnaire?" she asked.

"Of course," I said.

"I can write more if it will be helpful."

"We're all set." I smiled. "It will give us a starting point for the questions I'll ask you now."

We began discussing what had inspired Marjorie to call me. She had apparently been feeling bloated and was recovering from having a benign growth on her neck removed. As she was only in her early thirties, it was significant that she had experienced such a blockage. Her work as a film producer required her to travel back and forth between Los Angeles and New York on a regular basis, and she tended to favor spicy foods as well as acidic foods like tomatoes and oranges. We discussed her lifestyle.

"I saw on the questionnaire that you run."

"Yes."

"And participate in cycling events."

"Yes."

"And swim."

"Yes."

"And play basketball."

"Yes."

"And Pilates . . ."

"Yes. And I do yoga too."

"Right. Yoga. And you exercise five or six times per week?"

"Yup. About that. There are some weeks where I find myself doing something just about every day, though." She downed the last of her ice water. It was becoming clear to me what was causing Marjorie's health troubles.

· · ·

Jennifer sat across from me in her big comfy recliner and was silent for several moments before she answered my question. Her large, wide eyes were looking at me, and yet they didn't seem particularly focused.

"I guess I'm kind of confused," she said at last. "I don't really eat that much, because the tumors make it painful to eat. But I do snack a lot."

"I see," I said in response. "The tumors are leaning into the stomach, causing discomfort while you digest; is that correct?"

"That's what my doctor said, yes." She then remained silent for several more moments.

"I know I like to eat snacks, but still—why should I be so overweight? It's not like I eat that much."

I had noticed when I entered her home that her living room smelled of french fries, which she might have had the night before. She had few decorations, plants, or objects, but she did have piles of DVDs surrounding a large plasma-screen TV. A stereo in the corner was likewise surrounded by CDs, and between these items and the plush, comfortable furniture, she seemed to have created an environment centered on watching and listening. Her laptop was set up on a small table near the couch I was sitting on, with the screen facing the same direction as the TV. If she were to sit at that laptop, her view of the TV would be unobstructed. We were sitting in the heart of Manhattan, but the soft, dense energy of her apartment presented as sharp a contrast to the fast pace of the New York City streets as taking a trip to a farm in the country. She had written that her main reason for contacting me was because she had fibroid tumors on her uterus, which were a consistent source of pain.

"On your questionnaire you wrote how you eat a lot of cookies and candy, especially during the workday, right?"

She considered this for several moments. "That's right," she finally said, "but like I said, I don't eat that much at a time."

"You also wrote how you don't take any time to eat in quiet, and instead eat while watching TV or being on the computer."

"Yes," she said.

"Well, it is very hard for the mind and body to be operating on such a diet and lifestyle. Whenever our bodies start creating a condition like tumors, it's a sign that our current lifestyle isn't working and that we need to do something about it."

Her eyes progressed to a point several feet to the left of me and stayed focused on this point. She did, of course, already know this—even if she wasn't aware that she knew.

"Jennifer," I said, "what is it that you really want?"

Her eyes found mine once again. For one moment I had the sense that she was looking at me and seeing me at the same time.

"I don't want to be in pain anymore," she said.

"Good," I said. "Knowing that is a very good start."

"Do you think you can help me?" she asked.

"I think that, once you begin doing the work, everything is going to get better for you."

She considered this for several moments. Then she smiled.

. . .

Christina and I had discussed her background as well as her health issues and the general dryness she was feeling in her body. She worked as a travel journalist and was on the road at least eight months out of the year. She had found a lump on her breast for which she was seeing a specialist the following month, she was very constipated and only moved her bowels every few days, and she had been experiencing sciatica and other nerve problems for a number of years. All of this led to her having very interrupted or non-existent sleep. We had now moved on to discussing the various changes she could make in her lifestyle and how she could improve her health.

"The lump on your breast might be taken care of if you simply go on a fast for a week," I said. "It's worth trying before you do any more invasive treatments."

"Yes," Christina replied, "I don't eat very much anyway, so yes, I could do that."

"It will help you to rid yourself of toxins that have built up from all of the traveling you do for your job. But as you have a history of anorexia and bulimia, I will have to guide you on this fast on a day-to-day basis to see how your body reacts to the changes."

"Okay, that makes sense."

"You also wrote on your questionnaire that you're eating a lot of salads and other raw vegetables, hummus, and fiber bars," I said.

"Well sure, I'm trying to stay healthy." Her eyes started darting back and forth when she said this.

"Yes, while vegetables are good, and they say they put a lot of nutrients in those bars, the bars are very dry and the raw vegetables have a lot of air in them. It is important that you instead start eating cooked vegetables and cooked rice, and avoid the kinds of foods that come in packages, like the fiber bars. You'll also need to eat your food with natural oils, which you're currently not getting."

"Well, why does it matter about consuming oil?" she asked, now fidgeting with her hands while her eyes darted around the room. "Isn't water what's supposed to hydrate us?"

"Actually, while it's important to eat foods with high water content like fruits and vegetables, it's the consumption of oils that lubricates the system and will help you to no longer experience constipation and other forms of dryness."

"Do I have to find a different job or career or something?"

I stopped for a beat. "What do you mean?"

"Well, if traveling is so bad and toxic, do I have to find a different job that doesn't make me travel so much?"

I wasn't sure how Christina had jumped to that conclusion or why her mind had picked that one detail about travel out of everything we had discussed so far. She continued to fidget and shift in her seat.

"No, you certainly don't have to quit your job," I said, "as there are ways of incorporating these practices into your lifestyle."

"Oh. Good. I don't know what I would do without my job."

"Indeed. You'll be able to simply bring oils with you as you travel, and lean toward certain foods that keep more moisture in the body."

"Wait—why is moisture so important?" Shift, fidget, shift.

"I'm sorry?" I said.

"I'm not sure what moisture has to do with it, if you said I don't need to hydrate myself and don't need water." Fidget, fidget, shift.

"Well, it's not that you don't need water, it's that you're going to use oils to lubricate your organs and deeper tissue. Water is still very important."

"Right. It's just easier to drink water, that's all."

I sat there for a moment and watched her as she shifted about even more nervously.

"Perhaps," I said, "we should just breathe for a moment. I'll show you how."

"Yes, breathing," she said. "I can do that."

"Of course you can," I replied.

. . .

Each of these three women was suffering from some sort of ailment or condition that she was looking to resolve by working with me. Another thing you might have noticed is that each woman exhibited not only different kinds of symptoms and discomfort, but also different personality traits and behaviors.

Marjorie was feeling bloated, was aggressive with her hosting duties and unable to settle down until she had taken care of certain tasks, was incredibly active in her lifestyle, and was sweating even in an air-conditioned apartment on a mild day. In contrast, Jennifer spent much of her time watching TV or on the computer, took a long time to respond to or even focus on what we were talking about, was overweight, and had fibroid tumors that pushed up into her stomach area and inhibited her ability to comfortably digest food. Christina experienced dryness to the point of feeling constipated, was constantly fidgeting with nervous energy, and couldn't focus on the concepts we were discussing for more than a short period of time.

Each person received a different treatment plan and was asked to make different lifestyle changes. Each had filled out a questionnaire about her health and lifestyle prior to our meeting, and the questionnaires that these three women filled out are located in the back of this book as appendices A–C. The work that I did with these women is based on the ancient Indian medicinal system known as Ayurveda. Through exploring these women's stories and some basic practices, in this chapter I will guide you through Ayurvedic teachings and show how you can use these tools to restore balance in your life.

what is ayurveda?

Before Western medicine, before homeopathic medicine, and before even traditional Chinese medicine, there was Ayurveda, an ancient system of healing created by sages in India over five thousand years ago. While yoga was developed as a science for the practitioner to bring balance and control to the mind, Ayurveda is a sister science developed for the practitioner to bring balance to the body.

Western medicine tends to treat a patient's symptoms with different pills and medications without any attention to healing the cause of a disease that is feeding the symptom. It is like weeding a garden without taking out the roots; the weeds just grow back. Ayurveda works to define the cause of the patient's symptoms and to treat the body with various methods for the sake of restoring balance to the system as a whole. When that balance is attained, the body naturally frees itself of disease. It is for this reason that modern-day culture calls Ayurveda a holistic system of healing.

The first question that an Ayurvedic healer contemplates is, quite simply, what is the cause of these symptoms? In Christina's case, for example, a Western doctor might simply give her a stool softener or laxative and send her on her way. In contrast, an Ayurvedic healer deduces that her constipation and other conditions all relate back to one central imbalance in the body, which in this case is excessive dryness and movement of the body and mind. She needs to be put on a regimen that requires simple modifications to the diet, like the consumption of oils, and she also needs a change in sleeping habits. To use Ayurveda as a tool is to know oneself better, rather than complicating one's health with unnecessary remedies or asking doctors to tell us how we feel.

Through a precise, detailed system of observing what is occurring in the body, the Ayurvedic patient's diseases are diagnosed and treated with substances and routines that are already found in nature. The treatment plan that an experienced Ayurvedic healer might present to you is based on eating certain food groups, taking certain herbs, having certain treatments, and making certain modifications to your lifestyle, and this is how I approached working with the three patients described in this chapter. The purpose of this chapter is not only to introduce you to the concepts and theories behind Ayurveda, but also to provide you with a practical guide so you have the knowledge and ability to treat yourself for many common issues like constipation, digestive problems, insomnia, migraines, the flu, allergies, asthma, arthritis, obesity, and many others. You will likely be amazed at how simple and attainable it is for us to restore health and balance to our bodies when we make it a priority.

ayurveda and the five elements

Whether we're fans of fantasy role playing, science fiction movies starring Bruce Willis, or seventies R & B groups that sing about boogie wonderlands, most of us have heard of fire, water, earth, air, and ether, also known as the classical elements. These five entities are considered in various philosophical systems to be the fabric of all of life, and Ayurveda uses this system for assessing balance or imbalance in our bodies.

The ancient sages who developed Ayurveda many centuries ago observed that our bodies could be viewed as made up of these five elements. Each of us has fire or heat in the body; much of our bodies are made up of water; our organs and other vital components are made of dense matter like earth; we breathe in air; and there is abundant space—or ether—in between the cells that make up our being.

The metaphor, however, does not end with a mere comparison between the elements and body tissue. It also extends to three types of energies that sustain and determine the quality of our lives. One type of energy allows us to metabolize for the sake of processing oxygen and perpetuating life. Another type of energy forms our bodies, which serves as a container so that life can exist as matter. The third type of energy shifts matter's position in space through the act of motion. I mentioned that Ayurveda is the sister science to yoga and is intended to observe and treat the body. The ancient sages understood these three types of energy to form the fundamental reality of our entire physical existence.

However, they observed only three components of physical existence, and yet there are five elements. The sages determined that these three components were the product of grouping the five elements into pairs: fire with water, earth with water, and air with ether.

The sages saw that each of these three components manifests as a distinct energy type in the body, and that this energy is either in balance or not. They labeled each type as a *dosha,* or basic constitution. Each one of us is made up of some amount of all three constitutions.

- The *Pitta* dosha is comprised of the fire and water elements and represents the heat and fire in the body responsible for digesting food and breaking down toxins. Pitta energy sits mainly in the stomach and small intestines.

- The *Kapha* dosha is comprised of the earth and water elements and represents the dense, earthlike container that forms our bodies and helps root us. Kapha energy sits mainly in the head and chest region.

- The *Vata* dosha is comprised of the air and ether elements and is responsible for movement and elimination in the system. Vata energy sits mainly in the large intestine.

In Ayurveda, observing the relationship of these three doshas in our bodies is the basis of understanding our behaviors, creating and maintaining health, and, ultimately, determining the cause of our imbalances.

UNDERSTANDING THE ELEMENTS IN RELATION TO OUR PERSONALITIES

If you've already been introduced to Ayurveda through another book or a magazine article, you probably also learned about the doshas through the act of determining your dosha type. When introducing the science of Ayurveda, writers often put forward the idea that each of us is fundamentally Pitta, Kapha, or Vata in our constitution. An Ayurveda quiz is often included, which is a series of questions about your lifestyle and behaviors that helps you to identify your dominant dosha.

This practice is based on the idea that each of us has a constitutional dosha type that defines our mentalities and our physical attributes from the day we are born until the day we die. The quiz might tell us that we're a Kapha (earth) person or that we're mostly Pitta (fire). Most of us love learning about ourselves by taking quizzes, and it is certainly helpful to assess the condition of our bodies through such a process—but it is not conclusive. What often happens is that when we hear that we're "a predominantly Vata (air) personality," we attach ourselves to the idea that this is our nature—as fixed as the sum of two plus two.

My studies in India taught me otherwise. Each of us is born into this world with an abundance of one or two of the three doshic energies as influenced by our own mother's and father's elemental natures. The dominant energy we're born with may very well remain the most dominant energy throughout our lives. The misconception, though, is that it cannot change or will never trade places with one or two of the other energies.

For purposes of assessing health and balance, it is less significant what energy we were born with and more significant what energy we have in the present moment. Our current energetic state is defined by the decisions we make and the actions we take in the days, months, and years leading up to the moment in which we are assessing ourselves. For this reason I will never suggest to you that you're a "Pitta person" or a "Kapha person." I'll only suggest that you have an abundance or excessive amount of one or two of the three different types of energies. I too have included a quiz for self-assessment later in this chapter, but as all of us have all three energies, it is intended only to help you determine which energies are most out of balance at the present time. Oddly enough, the quiz often turns out to be more accurate if someone who knows us well fills it out for us, as we often are not able to see ourselves clearly.

Marjorie, the woman in the first story, had an abundance of Pitta energy. She committed a lot of hours to her job, took on a number of other activities in addition to her job, exhibited a compulsive need to complete the questionnaire in the proper way, ate spicy foods, and generated a lot of extra heat in her body. In contrast, Jennifer was much more lethargic and vegetative in her lifestyle and was experiencing an excess of heavy Kapha energy. In the third story, Christina was feeling scattered, anxious, and restless, which was indicative of her excessive Vata energy.

Each of these women's personalities and emotions was related to the excess of energy she was feeling, and through our consultation process it became apparent that these energies had been dominant throughout their lives. While I was curious about which type of energy each woman originally inherited from her parents, when it came to restoring balance to each of their lives, it was more important for me to learn about their current energetic state, which they can control.

The treatments outlined in this chapter are not intended to define how to relate to your body in one fixed way throughout the rest of your life but are intended rather to show you how to use your behaviors, lifestyle, environment, and ailments as indicators to help you determine which elements need to be brought into balance and therefore how to treat yourself at this point in time. Remember, our health is like the weather, forever moving and changing. It is our responsibility to adapt to those changes and control the one thing we can—our actions.

With all of this said, it is still helpful to observe how our personalities relate to the three doshic energies. What follows is an overview of the behaviors and emotions relating to each dosha.

- Our Pitta energy drives us to achieve, accomplish goals, and exhibit fiery qualities like passion and anger. When in balance, Pitta energy can help a person to remain focused, get things done, and maintain an active lifestyle. When excessive, Pitta energy can cause a person to heat up and feel angry, temperamental, and overpowering.

- Our Kapha energy helps us to feel grounded, facilitates our nurturing of others, and helps us exhibit a calming presence in stressful situations. When in balance, Kapha energy can help a person to relax, play the role of caretaker, and maintain a sense of stability. When excessive, Kapha energy can cause a person to feel heavy and lethargic, experience worry, and smother others.

- Our Vata energy helps us to explore creativity and inquisitiveness, express ourselves, and remain in motion. When in balance, Vata energy can help a person to remain open to change, explore new situations, and find alternative solutions to problems. When excessive, Vata energy can cause a person to feel scattered, nervous, and manic.

As you might imagine, the holistic nature of Ayurvedic medicine considers both how these energies affect our emotional state and how they affect our mental and physical health—as well as how these various aspects of our lives relate to each other. By observing both our bodies and our minds, we are able to use this system of the doshas to determine the cause of our imbalances.

UNDERSTANDING THE ELEMENTS IN RELATION TO OUR HEALTH

Modern medicine is under ninety years old, and those training to practice it spend many years growing their skill level and knowledge base. By contrast, Ayurveda is five thousand years old, with an accumulated knowledge base on how to attain health and longevity that spans many centuries.

This is a lot of information.

Though it would be useful to explain to you the many nuances of the Ayurvedic system as it relates to training Ayurvedic practitioners—how we have not just doshas but subdoshas, how we have different tissues and channels, and the many, many other components of this ancient science that are taken into account when exploring the question of health—I'm not going to attempt that here. The purpose of this chapter is instead to teach you basic facts about the process of restoring balance. With this information, you may make simple modifications to your lifestyle and enjoy harmony in the body.

All of us have the same energies in the body, but our habits and lifestyles determine what level of balance or imbalance we experience. Each energy can be aggravated out of balance, and if one energy is aggravated, it is likely that one or both of the other energies are diminished.

- *Pitta energy can either heat the body or burn it.* We use our Pitta energy to accomplish tasks and essentially metabolize our ability to soldier on. If we live with excessive heat in the form of constantly working, eating spicy foods, overexercising, indulging in excessive sex, and other forms of intense activity, then we'll likely aggravate our Pitta, or fire, energy. When this happens, our muscles might get inflamed, we might have liver complaints, we might experience indigestion and other issues of the gastrointestinal tract, and we might also experience bloating or fatigue.

- *Kapha energy can either ground the body or encumber it.* We use our Kapha energy to ground ourselves and ensure our physical stability. If we eat heavy foods, remain sedentary, and shirk our responsibilities in favor of vegging out, then we'll likely aggravate our Kapha, or earth, energy. When this happens, we might gain weight, develop diabetes, experience a stagnant mind, and feel a general sense of heaviness or of being stuck without any way to emerge from such lethargy.

- *Vata energy can either move the body or dry it.* We use our Vata energy to keep ourselves responsive to the ever-changing conditions of our lives. If we live in excessive motion in the form of eating cold foods, constantly traveling, and losing ourselves to an avalanche of thoughts in any given moment, then we'll likely aggravate our Vata, or air, energy. When this happens, we might have dry skin, suffer from insomnia, experience constipation and other conditions indicative of a dry system, and feel scattered and distracted when we set out to accomplish a task or understand an idea.

diagnosing imbalances

So how can we use this information to determine how to treat body complaints and disease? Earlier in the chapter I suggested that using Ayurveda to free ourselves of disease and create balance begins with investigating the cause of the imbalance. Ayurveda's diagnosis process centers on the fact that since we are made up of nature (the elements), we are to observe how our bodies are responding to the imbalances of nature in the form of food, the weather, or other living things. To remain in health, we must determine how the general order of our bodies is departing from an ideal natural state and moving toward dis-ease.

The most highly trained Ayurvedic doctors study for years with their gurus to gain the knowledge necessary to treat the more nuanced and complicated diseases of the body. While this system relies on a simple construct of three energy types to explain the body's imbalances, the diagnosis process itself depends on many different tools to determine the root cause. A practitioner uses the outside of the body as a map to the inside of the body, such as using the texture of the skin to determine if a person is dry from excessive Vata energy or oily from excessive Pitta or Kapha energy.

How does the outside of the body indicate what is happening on the inside of the body? Diagnosing a condition with the use of Ayurvedic science happens by observing irregularities on the surface of the body, talking with the patient about lifestyle and habits, and using touch to discover any complications or symptoms that may or may not be visible.

OBSERVING

When I met with Marjorie, I observed that she was sweating, had a red complexion, and was a little aggressive in her thoughts toward herself and others. I noticed that Jennifer was overweight, led a sedentary lifestyle, and moved slowly. Christina tended to shift back and forth in her seat, had a difficult time focusing on what we were discussing, and blinked a lot.

One of the most significant components of Ayurvedic diagnosis is observing how a person looks, acts, and communicates, as imbalances manifest in many ways. If the whites of our eyes are yellow, then there may be liver problems; a white coating or film on the tongue indicates toxins in the stomach, intestines, and other organs. People can seem calm, or they can seem nervous. They can appear present, or they can appear aggravated. They can behave in a comforting way, or they can be fraught with worry. Whichever it is, the balance or imbalance will show up in plain view on the surface of the body.

How can you use the act of observation to understand your own imbalances? You can consider each of the three doshas and use what we know about each of their excesses to determine if you are feeling an imbalance. Are you feeling warmer in your body or cooler? Are you feeling oily, average, or dry? Are you feeling light, or are you feeling heavy? Do you tend to be more static or more mobile? Observing basic sensations in a series of moments over the course of a day or week can provide a great deal of insight into which imbalances you might be experiencing in your body.

take the dosha quiz

Taking a quiz to help determine our doshic imbalances can help us make a general assessment of our current condition. What follows are twenty-one questions that are broken down into physical traits and mental traits. Each question has three possible answers, and as you take the quiz you can write down the letter of each answer on a separate sheet of paper. Answer each question with clarity in the moment. This is meant to reflect how you truly see yourself rather than how you want to be.

Physical Traits

1. How would you describe your bodily proportions?
   a. My body is medium-sized and symmetrical.
   b. My body is large and stocky.
   c. My body is thin and lanky.
2. How would you describe your body's frame?
   a. My body is muscular.
   b. My body is thick and solid.
   c. My body is thin with little fat.
3. How would you describe your joints?
   a. My joints tend to be loose.
   b. My joints are large and tend to be padded.
   c. My joints are weak and tend to crack.
4. What tastes are you more drawn to?
   a. I like to eat sweet, bitter, and astringent foods.
   b. I like to eat pungent, bitter, and astringent foods.
   c. I like to eat sweet, sour, and salty foods.
5. How would you describe your skin?
   a. My skin is soft and warm.
   b. My skin is oily and moist.
   c. My skin is dry and rough.
6. How would you describe your hair?
   a. My hair is fine and thin.
   b. My hair is thick and abundant.
   c. My hair is dry and brittle.
7. How would you describe your fingernails?
   a. My fingernails are pink and soft.
   b. My fingernails are wide and thick.
   c. My fingernails are brittle and cracked.
8. How would you describe your eyes?
   a. My eyes are reddish and sensitive.
   b. My eyes are white and wide open.
   c. My eyes are small and dry.
9. How would you describe your appetite?
   a. My appetite tends to be strong and excessive.
   b. My appetite tends to be low but consistent.
   c. My appetite changes depending on how I'm feeling.
10. How would you describe your digestion?
    a. My digestion tends to be efficient and accommodating of many different foods.

b. My digestion tends to be slow.

c. My digestion is often very delicate and disturbed by many foods.

11. How would you describe your stool?

    a. My stool tends to be loose and sometimes burns.

    b. My stool tends to be solid and heavy.

    c. My stool tends to be small and hard.

12. What sort of environment tends to cause you the greatest discomfort?

    a. I don't particularly like hot days.

    b. I don't particularly like wet and humid days.

    c. I don't particularly like cold days.

Mental Traits

13. How would you describe your general personality?

    a. I tend to be intelligent and efficient.

    b. I tend to be calm and patient.

    c. I tend to be creative and imaginative.

14. What happens to you when you're under a lot of stress?

    a. I tend to be irritable and bad-tempered.

    b. I tend to be lazy and lethargic.

    c. I tend to be nervous and anxious.

15. How would you describe yourself in conversations with others?

    a. I tend to be argumentative and challenging.

    b. I tend to be silent and slow to respond.

    c. I tend to be talkative and chatty.

16. How do you tend to focus on the completion of tasks?

    a. When completing a task, I tend to focus on details.

    b. When completing a task, I tend to focus on the big picture.

    c. I tend to have a short attention span and can't focus on any one task for long.

17. How would you describe your learning temperament?

    a. I tend to be sharp and have a thorough understanding of what I've learned.

    b. I tend to be slow to understand new information and concepts but retain them thereafter.

    c. I learn things quickly and then forget about them just as quickly.

18. How would you describe your friendships?

    a. My friendships tend to center on shared purposes and functions.

    b. My friendships are long-lasting and intimate.

    c. My friendships tend to change from one period of my life to the next.

19. How would you describe your sleep habits?

    a. I tend to sleep soundly for an average length of time.

    b. My sleep tends to be heavy, and it's difficult to wake up the next morning.

    c. My sleep tends to be light, and I'm prone to awakening in the night.

20. How would you describe your general energetic state?
    a. I tend to have purposeful, sometimes aggressive energy.
    b. I tend to have relaxed, sometimes leisurely energy.
    c. I tend to have frenetic, sometimes scattered energy.
21. How would you describe your emotional traits?
    a. I tend to feel angry, jealous, passionate, and fiery.
    b. I tend to feel attached, possessive, compassionate, and understanding.
    c. I tend to feel unpredictable, fearful, enthusiastic, and adaptable.

Once you've answered each of these twenty-one questions, add up how many a's, b's, and c's you have.

If you have more a's than b's or c's, then your most excessive dosha is your Pitta energy.

If you have more b's than a's or c's, then your most excessive dosha is your Kapha energy.

If you have more c's than a's or b's, then your most excessive dosha is your Vata energy.

If you have a lot of not just one but two letters, then there is a greater imbalance in both of those elements.

Once you've determined which dosha is most excessive, you can then begin to use the tips in this chapter and other resources to begin settling that energy down and bringing a greater sense of balance to your body and mind.

TALKING

One of the best tools an Ayurvedic healer has for treating a patient is listening to the patient talk about his or her feelings, thoughts, and behaviors. I spend time with each client going through the answers given on the questionnaire and listening as she or he informs me of daily habits and lifestyle patterns that I'm not able to observe. Receiving answers to questions forms a good part of the information that helps to properly diagnose one's imbalances.

Though you might not have a conversation with yourself out loud, you can certainly ask yourself the types of questions a trained healer might ask you so you have a precise means of determining some of your more significant imbalances. Below are some questions you can ask yourself, and in the next section you'll learn more about the ways you can modify your lifestyle to ensure that your answers to these questions will inform a healthier, more balanced life.

- When do I go to bed? Is it early or particularly late? Is it at the same time, or is it inconsistent from night to night?

- When do I last eat each night? How long does my food have to digest before I go to bed?

- What do I eat? Do I eat more natural, live foods, or are they processed or left over from other meals?

- What do I drink? Do I drink a lot of caffeinated beverages, alcohol, and soft drinks, or do I drink more water and herbal teas?

- What are my thoughts like? Are they repetitive, calm, anxious, or another quality?

- Do I worry and fret over things on a regular basis?

- Is my body open and supple or stiff?

- Do I talk a lot?

TOUCHING

Since the information we gather for diagnosis tends to be diverse and sophisticated, it is of utmost importance not to diagnose a significant condition without having complete information. Knowing the right kind of questions to ask comes from having the necessary training and experience to know the significance of various details. A person's eyes right after crying are redder or drier than they are in general, thus leaving the possibly false impression that there is an excess of fire in the system. A person's tongue right after eating may have a color or filminess that isn't usually there.

One of the most significant diagnostic tools for a trained Ayurvedic healer is reading the patient's pulse. The rhythm, frequency, and intensity of the pulse can reveal if a person is experiencing an imbalance in one or more of the three doshas or organs and is a significant tool for drawing these conclusions. However, the pulse is also a good example of an indicator that a lay practitioner is unlikely to acquire reliable information from. You could check your pulse right after running, eating, sleeping, or sex and draw inaccurate conclusions about what is happening inside your body. It is important to note, however, that to read the pulse accurately takes many years of continuous practice.

When drawing conclusions about your own imbalances, it is best to rely on a more basic sense of touch. You can determine what your skin feels and looks like. If it is oily, there may be a Pitta or Kapha imbalance; if it is dry, there may be a Vata imbalance. You can also tell if parts of your body feel hot (Pitta) or cold (Vata), if parts of the body such as the joints feel inflamed, or if the stomach, head, or other parts feel imbalanced in any way.

living the ayurveda way

If you were to consult with an Ayurvedic therapist, you would likely receive a diagnosis of your doshic imbalances based on the tools described above. The practitioner would then provide you with a list of food types that you should and shouldn't eat, possibly prescribe medicinal herbs for you to take, prescribe treatments, and provide a series of other lifestyle modifications and routines such as yoga postures for you to practice.

Ayurvedic science calls upon us to live our lives in a particular way with the intention of bringing as much balance to our doshas as possible. Much of this lifestyle centers on how and what we eat and drink, as one of the most fundamental components of Ayurvedic science states that a strong digestion leads to a healthy body. While we can make sophisticated modifications of diet and lifestyle to resolve imbalances of our doshas, it is more important to understand the attributes of food (hot-cold, dry-oily, heavy-light, and so forth) and what effect they will have on our systems in the moment. In this section I will share with you general measures we can all take that can be practiced regardless of how our doshas are imbalanced, and the following section will provide very basic and simple ways to resolve issues specific to each dosha.

REGULATE YOUR TIME AND FREQUENCY OF EATING

In the Western culture, eating has become a way not just to sustain life and metabolize energy, but also to build social contacts and dampen or heighten our more difficult emotions. We may spend hours having dinner with friends, and because the event lasts for hours our food intake lasts for hours. When we're home alone, we may not feel particularly hungry on any given evening, but because we're bored while we're zoning out in front of the TV, we just feed ourselves to keep our mouths busy.

Keeping ourselves in balance, according to Ayurveda, centers on how and what we eat. This is because the food we eat becomes us, and balancing our doshas can begin with eating food for the sake of living rather than for the sake of our emotions or our social calendars. An Ayurvedic eating schedule is determined by what time it is best to digest food and what dosha we need to balance or avoid aggravating.

This schedule begins with not eating anything when we first wake up but instead waiting several hours for the digestive fire to build itself up, although people with a lot of Vata energy can tolerate a little food at that time. Rather than eating small amounts frequently, eat no more than two or three times during the day, with the final meal in the late afternoon or early evening. As Ayurvedic medicine believes that good health is based on strong digestion, it sees constantly eating as the root of most modern diseases. This habit makes the system work overtime and therefore creates an excess of toxic waste. In turn, cleaning out this waste requires more energy and at the same time creates an imbalance in the blood and all other organs. As it can take as much as ten hours to completely digest some foods, eating later than 5:00 or 6:00 p.m. means that the food will sit in the stomach while you sleep and will go to waste or turn to fat. Foods with little water content, like meat, will take even longer to digest and are best avoided in the latter half of the day. When you follow this routine, you will wake up less stiff in the morning, have more energy throughout the day, and crave more satisfying natural experiences in each and every moment with people who enhance your life.

EAT FOODS GROWN LOCALLY AND IN SEASON

If you were to go into the produce section of a supermarket, you would likely see an immense variety of fruits and vegetables. You might get strawberries from Chile in February or have year-round access to bananas from who knows what tropical environment. It has become a staple of our culture to have access to many different types of fruits and vegetables at all times. How, though, do these items find their way to our local supermarket? Between the time they have been grown in another part of the country or world and the time they arrive at your local supermarket, they have been harvested, packaged, shipped by boat or plane, transported by truck or train, and delivered on a flat along with other items. This arduous process subjects the foods to many different kinds of environments and makes it less nutritionally potent. As produce has to arrive on our plates looking good, it is picked prematurely, before it has ripened, and does not contain the potency of fresh products. It is like taking a baby away from its mother before it has all it needs to take care of itself. Hence, we have to overeat to receive the proper amount of nutrition from food.

Eating this type of food is toxic to the body, as our systems are not acclimated to the weather in the region where the food originated. For example, eating tropical fruits in the dead of winter puts unnecessary pressure on the digestive power. If, in addition to that pressure, we were to also have the flu, then the body's inability to support the ailment while also digesting difficult foods would lead to disease.

Visit local farmers' markets and other organic venues to buy your produce and other types of foods. This means that you might not have the same variety of foods at your disposal year-round, but you will ensure that the foods you do put in your body don't build up toxins and increase the risk of serious illnesses like cancer.

AVOID PROCESSED FOODS

For thousands of years, humanity lived on fresh fruits, vegetables, grains, and various animal proteins. People hunted, gathered, and grew everything they ate. Many survived on only fruits. They ate what they needed to survive and spent much of their time procuring that food. Humanity developed technology to aid the growing and harvesting of the various foods that were eaten and found ways to minimize the amount of time required to grow enough sustenance for all.

Then, humanity invented cheese doodles.

Humanity also invented chocolate chip cookies. And ice cream. And chocolate bars. And macaroni and cheese that can be microwaved in under a minute. And yogurt that fits into a tube so that a child can eat it while running off to a friend's house to try out the latest video game console. The list goes on. Since the industrial revolution, we have developed new and different ways to process our foods to make them more immediately gratifying and easier to prepare regardless of their nutritional value. Instead of following natural habits, we are making artificial and convenient junk food so we can continue living our ego-driven excessive lifestyles. We are bringing children into the world and feeding them this junk and wondering why they have behavioral problems. Many snacks can have up to twenty ingredients that are hard to pronounce, and some bags of potato chips don't even list potatoes as the first ingredient. As so many books and magazine articles have already stated, processed foods are detrimental to our health and should be avoided as much as possible.

This is not to say that junk food is evil. It simply isn't food. It is only a gap filler, lacking the nutrition to sustain a natural and healthy life. Because it is devoid of natural nutrition, we need to eat a lot more of it to survive. If we eat in excess, then we tax our systems and can't live in balance. We must therefore work toward eating foods with no more than four or five ingredients, as having more than that increases the chance that the food isn't natural. Also, avoid frozen food, leftovers, food prepared in the microwave, canned food, and other foods that have a diminished or nonexistent nutritional value. Food should be eaten not just for survival but for living a healthy and prosperous life.

AVOID COOKING IN OIL

In our culture it is popular to fry, sauté, or roast foods in oil. Why wouldn't it be? Many people find food cooked in oil to be very tasty. However, cooking food in oil heats the food to a point that destroys its nutritional value and builds up carcinogens that have been found in the Western world to cause cancer and add to obesity. Ayurvedic science shares this view and attributes many of the imbalances that have developed in the West to the abundance of foods cooked in oil.

However, this is not to say that we shouldn't consume oil. Quite the contrary. Oil is an important part of keeping the body well lubricated for proper digestion and elimination. Instead of cooking foods in oil, though, it is good to cook with water (steam) and then add the oil after the food is cooked. There are many beneficial oils, but a few more potent ones are: sesame oil (for Vata), coconut oil (for Pitta), and mustard oil (for Kapha). Olive, flaxseed, and sunflower are also good oils.

DRINK HOT WATER

Another staple of modern life is to drink icy cold beverages throughout the day. The body, as we all know, maintains a temperature of nearly 100 degrees Fahrenheit. The digestive fire must exist at a comparable level of heat to be able to function well. When we consume these icy beverages, be it water or another item like soda or beer, the digestive fire not only must perform its normal duties, it must also assimilate the beverage into the body's overall temperature. This weakens the fire, which means that food is not completely digested. With this weaker fire, we experience gastrointestinal issues like indigestion, constipation, acidity, and headaches.

The best way to avoid diluting the digestive fire is to favor hot or room-temperature water as the primary beverage of choice over soft drinks, alcohol, or ice water. Even people with an abundance of heat in the body because of a Pitta imbalance would benefit from favoring hot water over cold, as the extra work involved in consuming the cold beverages exacerbates the issues related to excessive heat.

AVOID DRINKING TOO MUCH DURING MEALS

We often like to wash our food down with a nice beverage. Consuming too much liquid while eating, however, puts out the digestive fire, much as water puts out a fire in the outside world and hampers it from burning as efficiently as it should. This leads to problems in a similar way that drinking cold beverages does. If you are inclined to drink beverages while eating, favor hot water or ginger tea over other choices as much as possible. During the meal, sip on your water and drink only enough to help digestion. If you feel full or bloated, however, you have drunk too much. Excess Vata energy will require more water, Pitta a little less, and Kapha very little.

REGULATE YOUR SLEEP

Ayurveda assigns doshic energy qualities not only to our bodies and minds, but also to certain times of the day. Each time of day is thought to be of a quality of either Pitta, Kapha, or Vata. Between about 2:00 and 6:00 in the morning tends to be Vata, between 6:00 and 10:00 a.m. is

Kapha, and from 10:00 a.m. to 2:00 p.m. is Pitta. The cycle then repeats, with 2:00 p.m. beginning the next Vata cycle, and so on.

Why is this significant? If we wake up at 4:00 or 5:00 a.m. during the Vata cycle, we are ensuring the greatest chance for activity and motion for the rest of the day. The evening Kapha cycle lasts from 6:00 p.m. to 10:00 p.m., so it is suggested that we go to bed by 10:00 p.m. when the more relaxing and calming Kapha energy is most prominent and will aid in sleep. If we regulate our sleep to wake up and go to sleep at consistent times and also to use these doshic guidelines, then we create a greater opportunity for balance and peace in our bodies and minds.

AVOID HEATING THE HEAD

Whenever we go into saunas and other environments of extremely high temperature, we're creating a lot of heat in the head. Given that our bodies exist at a certain temperature, applying such large amounts of heat to the head creates an excess of Pitta energy and thus adds anger and fear to the mind. It is best to avoid such extreme forms of heat like saunas, hot sunshine, and exercises like Bikram yoga so as to ensure balance, calm, and peace as we go through the day. As noted above in our discussion of violence, any extreme environmental condition challenges our bodies to maintain equilibrium and causes disharmony. Extreme heat also challenges our bodies to maintain the proper amount of digestive fire.

treating dosha imbalances

Marjorie began to sweat in an air-conditioned apartment. Jennifer snacked on a lot of unhealthy foods yet wasn't very hungry. Christina couldn't sit still for more than a minute. Each of these women was experiencing an aggravation of a particular dosha. Ayurvedic health practices center on bringing the doshas into balance and maintaining that balance, which is done not just by practicing the various components of health we just talked about but also by doing things to target specific doshas.

As I've already mentioned, however, it is important for a lay practitioner to make cautious use of the more sophisticated tools in this system. As the elements are continuously in motion, it is important for us to remain flexible in our lifestyles. If Marjorie were to correctly diagnose herself as having an excessive amount of Pitta energy, she might decide that she needs to never again eat tomatoes and acidic foods, never again eat spicy foods, and never exercise again. Though this might help her to settle the heat associated with her Pitta imbalance in the short term, over time it would likely push another dosha out of balance. For instance, the absence of exercise could create the heavy lethargy associated with excessive Kapha energy. Most people will always have more of not just one but two doshic energies, as a person who has more of only one is usually suffering from an extreme sickness or disease. It is when that energy is so low or exaggerated that disease settles into the body. For these various reasons, I encourage you to consult with an experienced practitioner to diagnose and treat more significant imbalances, and I will provide here only gentle ways for you to move your doshas in specific directions.

TREATING PITTA IMBALANCES

We might determine that we have a Pitta imbalance if we, like Marjorie, always feel hot, sweat profusely, have a reddish complexion, have blood in the stool, have red eyes, have gas, acidity, and other digestive issues, and consistently feel burned out from emotions of anger, hate, or aggravation. What follows are several ways we can settle excessive Pitta energy, including diet, a special posture sequence, and a specific breathing technique.

Cooling Pitta Energy with Food and Drink

Earlier in the chapter, I noted that Pitta energy can either heat the body or burn it. Through our consultation, I learned that Marjorie was experiencing a general sense of hotness in the body, which led to blood in the stool, gas, and even feeling hungry all day. I suggested these changes to bring Marjorie's Pitta energy into balance:

- Abstain from alcohol and other stimulants like caffeine, as they make the blood more acidic and hot. Avoid sour, salty, and pungent foods because they aggravate the Pitta dosha.

- Do not eat heavy foods like bananas, beef, lentils, and cheese for some time, as the more demanding digestion of these foods will aggravate the digestive fire. Spicy foods aggravated the digestive fire as well.

- Dissolve fennel, cumin, and coriander powders in hot water, and drink as a tea a few times a day to settle stomach acidity and build digestive strength. In the following chapter, I'll describe in fuller detail how to use herbs in this and other ways.

- Move toward a light diet, and eat only two times a day so the digestion can become strong again and the body can cool down a little.

These basic guidelines of abstaining from acidic, spicy, sour, and heavy foods, taking certain herbs, favoring lighter foods, and eating only twice a day can help you to resolve your excessive Pitta energy.

A Posture Sequence for Excessive Pitta Energy

Posture practice naturally opens the body, and it can also be used therapeutically to create more balance in the body and mind. Pitta energy, for example, can be settled through practicing less aggressive and fiery sequences than what are found in Ashtanga, Bikram, power yoga, or the practice usually taught in gyms. A person with excessive Pitta energy will want to cool the body and create more calm in the mind, and this is much more likely to happen with less aggressive systems of posture like restorative yoga, Hatha yoga, Kripalu yoga, and the following sequence.

For instruction on how to practice these postures, you can view videos of the sequence on my Web site or consult one of the many books available on posture. The postures in this sequence will encourage you to find greater balance and to focus on the moment. This sequence can be used to resolve Pitta-related complaints such as digestive issues, acidity, liver problems, ulcers, hypertension, thyroid problems, colitis, and excessive anger and aggression.

.   .   .

Visit yogicameron.com to view videos that will accompany the sequences for excessive Pitta, Kapha, and Vata energy.

tree

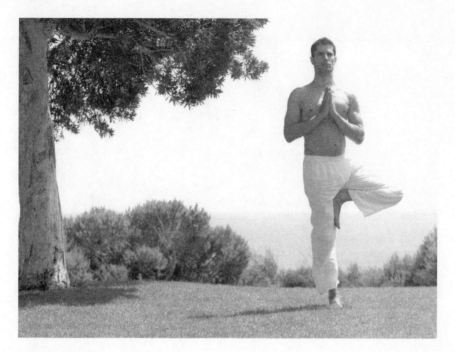

half moon

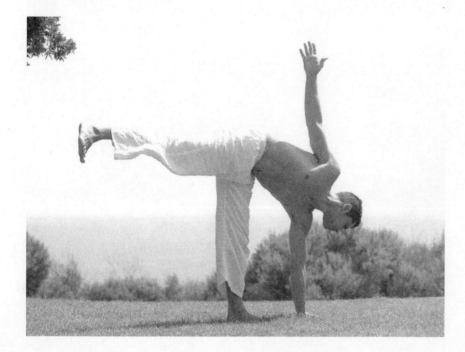

half shoulder stand

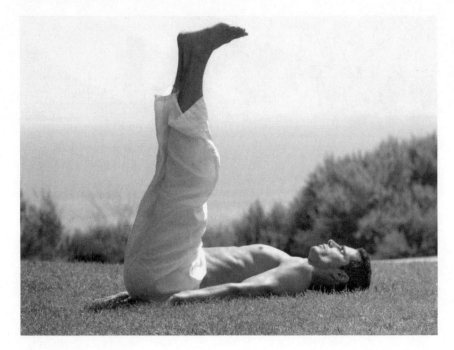

knee to chest

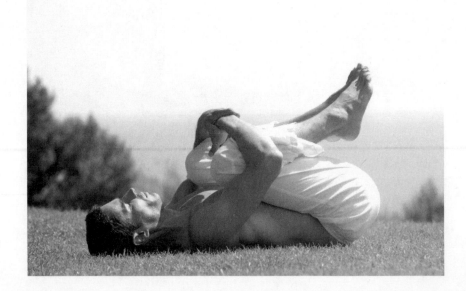

ear to knee

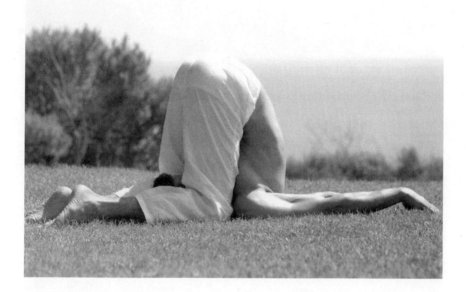

half bow

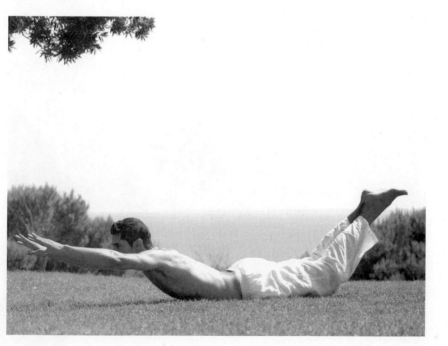

child's pose

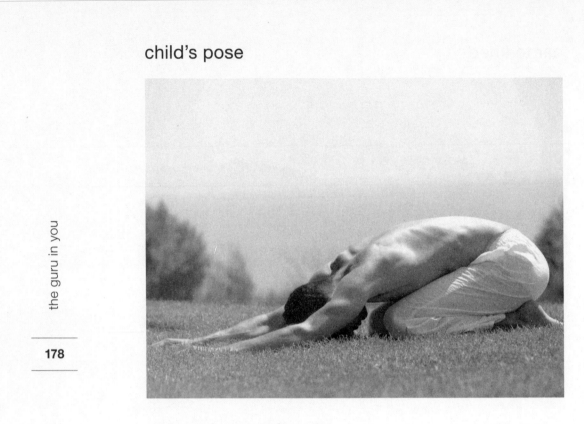

seated forward bend

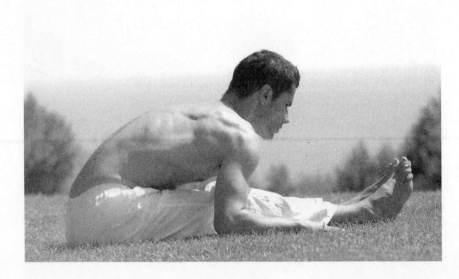

half twist

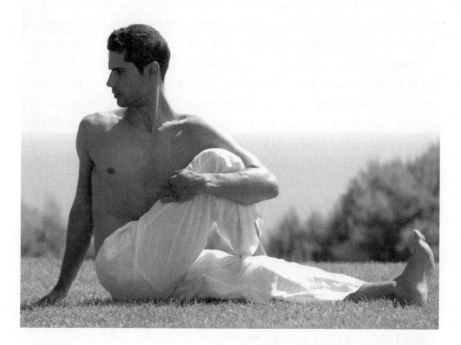

corpse

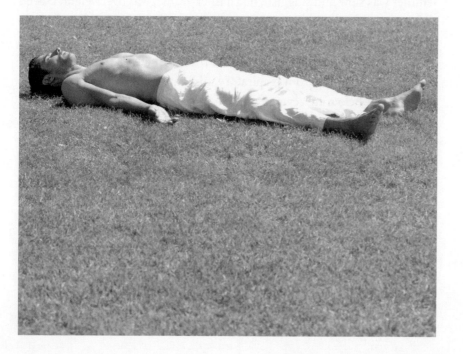

Breathing for Excessive Pitta Energy

Practicing alternate nostril breathing (see the previous chapter) will help to settle the mind regardless of our energetic imbalances, but we can use Ayurvedic science to affect our breathing practice in a more nuanced way.

Ayurveda and yogic science considers the right side of the body to consist of warmer, more masculine energy, and the left side home to a cooler, more feminine energy. If we are feeling excessively hot from an abundance of Pitta energy, we have an opportunity to breathe in only through the left nostril and out through the right nostril, which is half of the full alternate nostril breathing exercise. This is known as "moon breathing," as feminine energy is often associated with the cool nature of the moon in contrast to the warmer nature of the sun.

To help settle excessive Pitta energy, arrange your fingers as you did to practice alternate nostril breathing, close the right nostril, breathe in through the left nostril, close the left nostril, and breathe out through the right nostril. Repeat this until a cooling, calming sensation overtakes the body.

TREATING KAPHA IMBALANCES

Jennifer was slow and sluggish, had a thick frame, was overweight, craved a lot of sweet foods, felt drowsy in the morning, never exercised, and sat a lot. Jennifer and those of us who have Kapha imbalances feel excessively congested and filled with mucus, suffer from diabetes, suffer from throat problems, and suffer from respiratory ailments like bronchitis, sinusitis, and asthma. Below are several ways we can settle excessive Kapha energy.

Moving Kapha Energy with Food and Drink

Kapha energy can either ground the body, or it can encumber it. Jennifer felt a heaviness and lethargy that perpetuated her craving of sweet food and led her to compulsively snack all day, and she experienced issues with her digestion. I made these suggestions to help her balance her excessive Kapha energy:

- Refrain from eating sweet, sour, and salty tasting foods like cookies and chips, as they are not very nutritious and can cause weight gain.

- Refrain from talking on the phone or watching TV while eating, as the mindlessness of this eating habit can lead to excessive food consumption.

- Use ginger, cardamom, fennel, turmeric, and pepper to aid digestion.

- For a while, try eating once or at most twice a day, as the constant eating can create excess heat in the body—and a Kaphalike lack of activity can create energy blockages in response to that heat.

- Eat at 10:00 a.m., which is a more Pitta time, to have better digestion and avoid the earthy, heavier time of the early morning.

If you abstain from overindulging in Kapha-producing foods, limit your eating to only a couple of times a day, and bring greater mindfulness to your eating, you will be well on your way to restoring excessive Kapha energy. Developing willpower, as discussed in chapter 5, is also beneficial.

A Posture Sequence for Excessive Kapha Energy

A person with excessive Kapha energy will benefit from moving the body. Excessive Kapha energy can be resolved by practicing postures that require greater amounts of energy and by moving in more rapid succession from one posture to the next. This more energetic practice will help to move the heaviness of the Kapha energy, which in turn will facilitate the burning of excess fat and opening of the channels.

The postures in the following sequence encourage you to move with greater energy, but do not be forceful or competitive. I recommend you practice these postures for shorter durations of time, but repeat the sequence more than once. Be aware that as the body is feeling heavier and may not be flexible or agile enough to move around quickly, avoid any straining or overextending in postures. You may also notice that this posture doesn't end with corpse, as people with excessive Kapha energy tend to fall asleep in that posture. It is better instead to foster alertness by sitting to finish the practice. This sequence can be used to help resolve ailments in the head and chest areas, including asthma, sinusitis, sinus headaches, bronchitis, and throat problems, as well as diabetes, and the traits of laziness, possessiveness, and attachment.

downward-facing dog

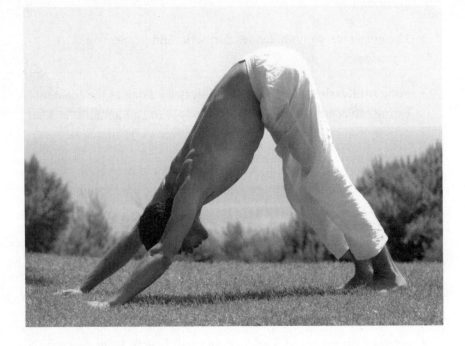

upward-facing dog

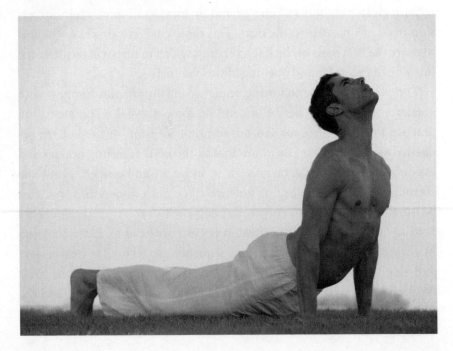

warrior 2

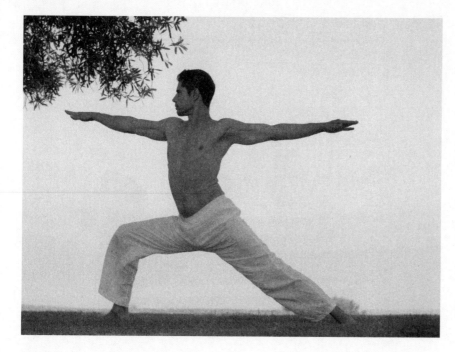

fish

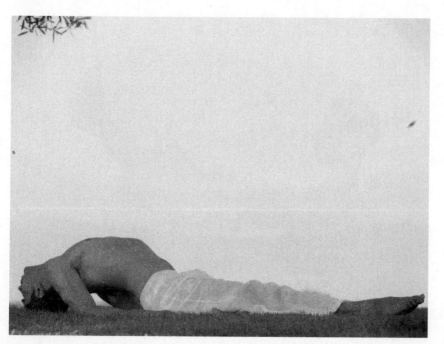

living the ayurveda way

bow

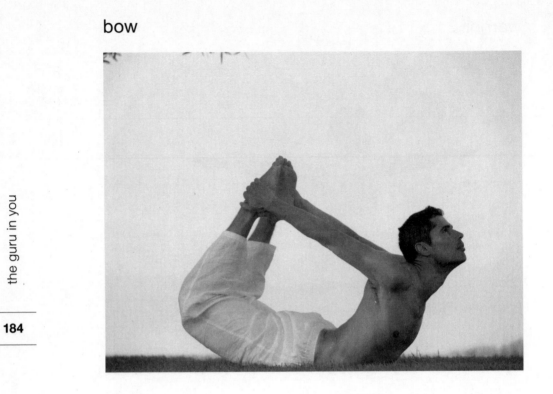

boat

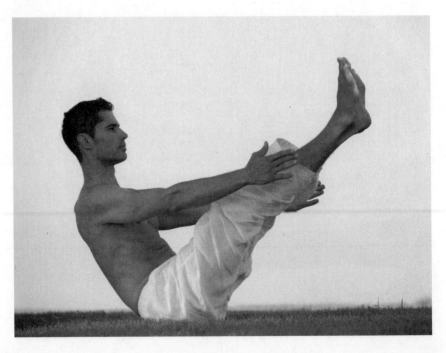

plow

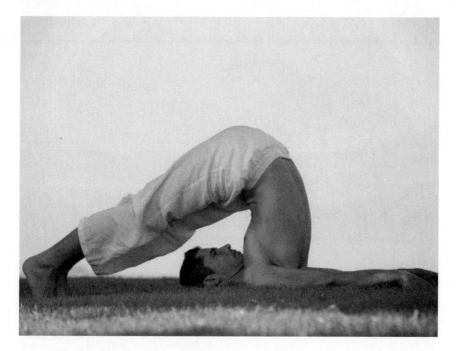

forward bend

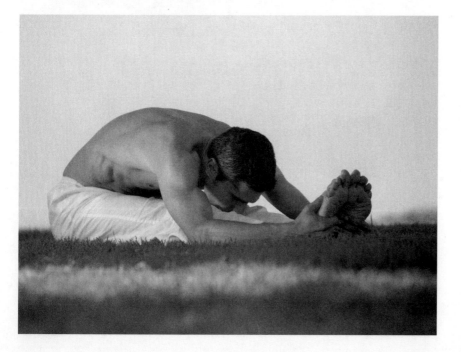

backward bend

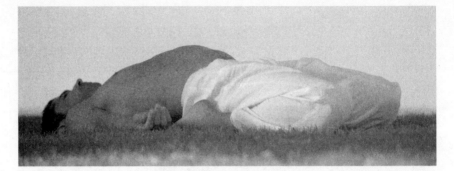

easy pose (seated posture)

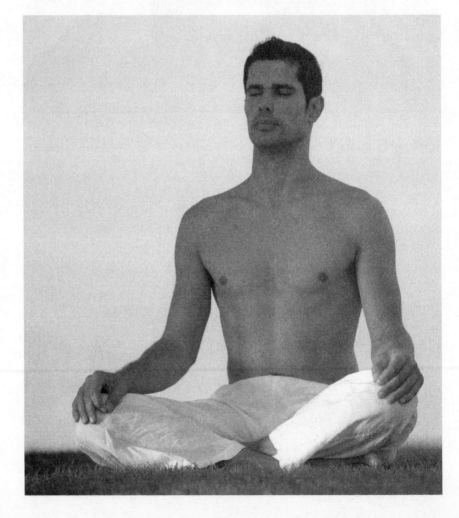

Breathing for Excessive Kapha Energy

If we are feeling excessively heavy from an abundance of Kapha energy, we can do the reverse of the technique used for diminishing the heat of excessive Pitta energy and breathe in through the right nostril and out through the left nostril.

Arrange your fingers as you did for alternate nostril breathing, close the left nostril, breathe in through the right nostril, close the right nostril, and breathe out through the left nostril. Repeat this as many times as you find appropriate.

breath of fire

Breath of fire is a commonly used breathing technique, but when I began studying it was not a daily part of my practice for one simple reason: I didn't need to create more heat in my body. Breath of fire earns its name from the fact that practicing it builds a lot of heat in the body. It is common for yoga teachers to incorporate this practice into their Vinyasa and power yoga classes, even if the students have little need for additional—or any—heat. If you have an abundance of Kapha energy, however, more heat will be of benefit to you.

1. From a seated position, take several full breaths.

2. After exhaling a full breath completely, take in a breath about three-quarters of the way through the nostrils, and forcefully push out the air through the nostrils by sucking in the abdomen rapidly.

3. Repeat this action continuously, pausing for a second between repetitions. This allows the stomach to rest and be ready for the next breath.

4. Continue this practice, beginning with about one breath per second and then quickening the pace as you become more adept.

5. There is no need to think of inhaling, as it happens naturally. Focus only on sucking in the abdomen and expelling the air.

6. To end the practice, slow the pace down, and then take several full breaths once again.

When learning this technique, it should not be practiced for more than a minute, and it should be avoided if you have high blood pressure or heart problems. Please see my Web site for a video demonstration of how this technique is practiced.

TREATING VATA IMBALANCES

Christina had particularly dry skin, suffered from insomnia, had a hard time sitting still or focusing on anything for a lengthy period of time, had chronic lower back pains, and suffered from bad constipation. If you suffer from a similar variety of conditions, then it is likely that you have excessive amounts of Vata energy in your body. What follows are several ways we can settle excessive Vata energy.

Settling Vata Energy with Food and Drink

Vata energy can either move the body and fluids or dry them. Christina was excessively thin and ate only a few limited types of food, including dry items like crackers and fiber bars. I suggested she make these dietary changes:

- To lubricate the body, use ghee (clarified butter) in cooking and in food. Ghee is an essential part of a balanced diet. Try consuming greater amounts of other oils like sesame. This can help the process of elimination return to normal and balance the digestion.

- Refrain from consuming crackers, fiber bars, and alcohol, as these dry out the body further.

- Consume herbs like licorice, saffron, clove, aloe vera, and gotu kola to bring a more grounding, Kaphalike energy to the system.

- Apply sesame oil to the outer body as the skin and muscles need more nutrition and lubrication.

These basic guidelines of consuming more oils, abstaining from dry foods, and consuming certain herbs can help you to resolve your excessive Vata energy.

A Posture Sequence for Excessive Vata Energy

People with excessive amounts of Vata energy can't help moving a lot and will therefore benefit from grounding the body. Excessive amounts of Vata energy can be resolved by spending greater amounts of time in each posture. This will help you to build your ability to stay still and be present in both body and mind.

The postures in this sequence will encourage you to move less and spend more time in the present moment. Spend some time in each pose, especially if you feel eager to move. This sequence will help you to resolve constipation, back pain, dryness and roughness of the skin, arthritis, sexual debility, insomnia, menstrual irregularities, and the traits of depression and anxiety.

tree

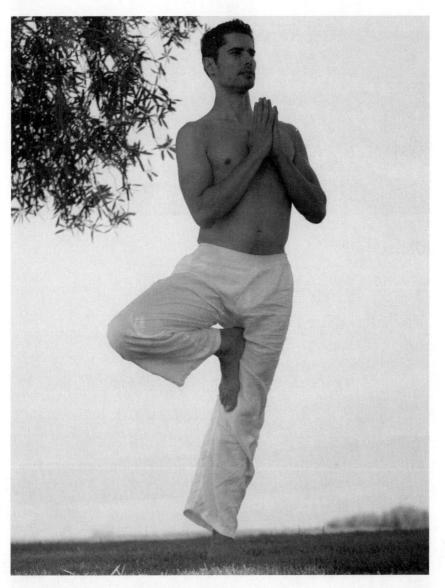

half shoulder stand

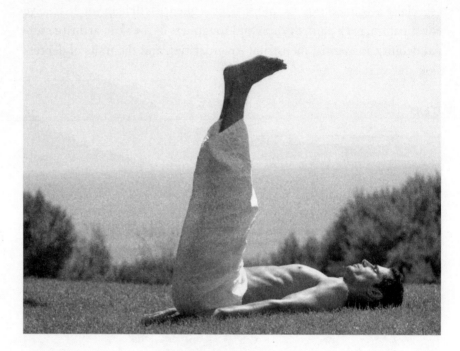

locust

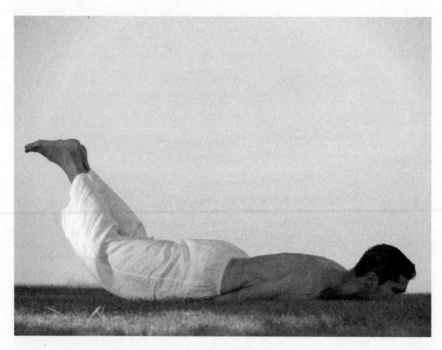

head to knee with knee bent into thigh

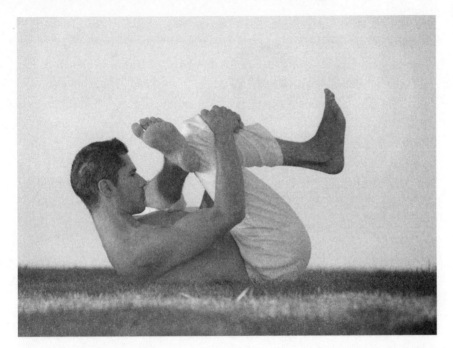

child's pose

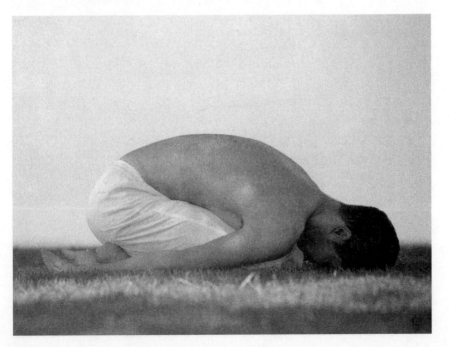

spinal twist

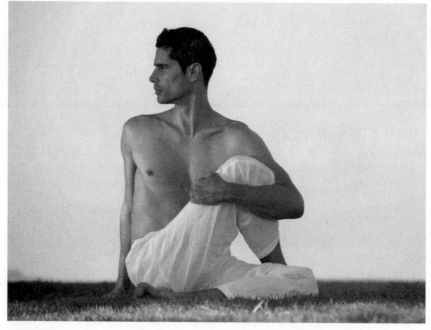

plow

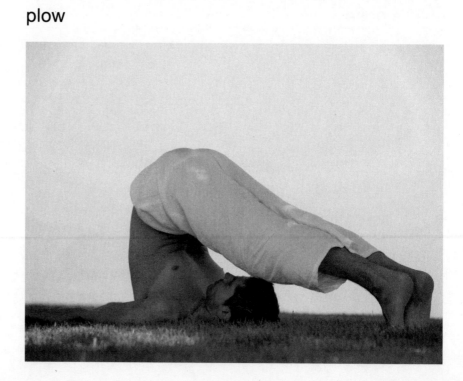

half wheel / bridge

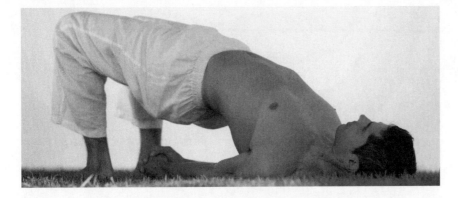

hero's pose

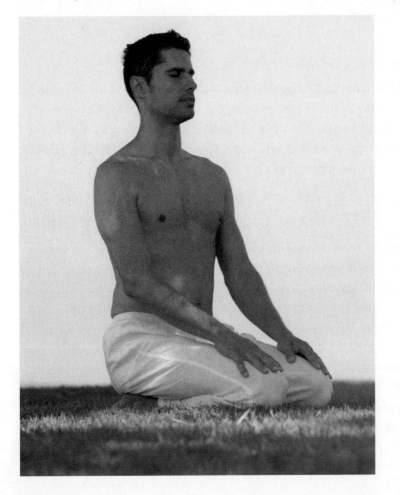

living the ayurveda way

corpse

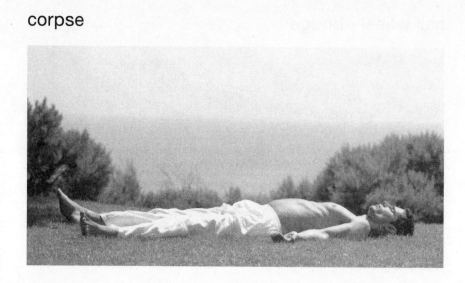

Breathing for Excessive Vata Energy

To settle Vata energy, it's best to use the alternate nostril breathing technique as outlined in the previous chapter. Breathing through both nostrils creates energy in both the male and female energy polarities, which helps the Vata energy to settle down. Repeat the steps of this exercise as many times as you find appropriate.

· · ·

Early results from Marjorie, Jennifer, and Christina were as expected. Marjorie cooled herself down, resolved her digestive issues, and no longer had blood in her stool. Jennifer lost weight and reduced the size of her tumors so that she could eat without experiencing any pain or discomfort. Christina began having regular bowel movements and getting a solid night's sleep. The fact that these results occurred is a testament to how their commitment to living the Ayurvedic way brought them greater balance and health. However, these changes represented only the beginning. If the goal of their practice was to gain balance, then reversing the changes they made to their lifestyles would reverse these short-term results as well.

When using Ayurveda to bring yourself into balance, there is much more to learn in addition to the material in this chapter. Instead of reading one book on Ayurveda after another, though, consider simply experimenting for some time with the various tools offered in these pages and find out what happens when you live the Ayurveda way yourself. I can share theories, facts, and practices with you, but the best way to learn about Ayurveda is to give it a try and observe how you feel.

The three women whose stories appear here began to make changes and experience positive results. Whether or not you join them in beginning to make lifestyle changes, however, is entirely up to you.

fill in the blank

Living the Ayurveda way can be a significant undertaking if done all at once. To begin making this lifestyle an integral part of your life, take the dosha quiz and then pick several of the tasks outlined in this chapter to try out—be it ridding your home of processed foods or having a dosha-specific tea in response to the results of the quiz—and live this way for several days before moving on to chapter 9.

9 practices for building awareness

YOU PROBABLY ALREADY KNOW that there is a great deal of information available on practices related to yoga and Ayurveda beyond the scope of this book. The chapters in this book provide just a sample of practices available in the yogic and Ayurvedic traditions, and yet these practices could keep the devoted practitioner busy for months or even years. However, there are other ways to explore and support one's practice in this tradition.

This chapter provides a sampling of other ways to build your practice and foster greater awareness of yourself in your path toward balance and joy. Some subjects are more practical in nature while others are more conceptual. Each one provides you with an opportunity to supplement the practices outlined in the earlier chapters of the book. You may very well find, though, that the first eight chapters have given you plenty of practices to work on for some time.

concentration

I encounter many people in the West who speak of what they call their "meditation practice." This practice usually involves sitting for certain periods of time trying to focus the mind on counting, repeating certain words to themselves, or some other technique. However, it is a misconception to consider these various techniques to be different forms of meditation. *Meditation* is the act of holding a conscious awareness that is entirely absent of thought. It is taught as a more advanced practice than the counting or word-based techniques commonly thought of as meditation, and it takes years of long, dedicated, daily practice to attain. The practice so many of us perceive to be meditation is actually the practice of *concentration*.

Let's say your job at work is to manage a series of accounts at an advertising agency. You're required to be a liaison between the creative team, the production team, and the clients and to make sure that all related groups are successfully collaborating to create content. In any given day you receive a dozen phone calls and two dozen e-mails, and four or five people stop by, supposedly to ask you about a PowerPoint presentation you're putting together but really just wanting to show you pictures of their fabulous vacations in Fiji. Though you tout yourself as an expert multitasker, you can't help but feel that each time you switch your focus from one task to another, you're not giving any one of them your full attention. By the end of the day, you get some of your work done, but the scattered quality of your attention has precluded you from feeling any real sense of accomplishment. The most consistent byproduct of all of your work, in fact, is likely to be a migraine from trying to focus on too many things in a short period of time.

This is how our minds work. The many different thoughts that come in and out of the brain in any given moment ultimately lead us to not remain focused on any one idea or thought for very long at a time. Just as the e-mail you were writing or the presentation you were finishing is only a marginal reflection of your ability, these many scattered thoughts are only a marginal reflection of your intelligence and spirit. Not only that, but we react to each thought we have and burden ourselves with stressful sensations in the body. In the middle of working on a task, we might think of what we would like to have for dinner that night. This creates an emotion ("Wow! I'm totally excited to have pad thai for dinner, and it's going to be great!"), and this emotion stimulates the senses. Our stimulated senses then induce attachments and more desires. When our senses are stimulated, our breath is thrown out of balance. And as we explored, having an imbalanced breath leads to an imbalanced life.

Concentration, and eventually meditation, fosters our ability to focus more deeply on each individual moment. The practice consists of giving the mind one thing to focus on instead of the many thousands of other things flitting in and out throughout the day. Building a greater sense of concentration not only will help to bring greater balance to the mind and body, but it also will play a significant role in improving our competence and contentment in any task we try to accomplish.

silence

I've known people to wake up in the morning, turn on the morning television news show in the bedroom as they figure out what they're wearing to work, turn on the radio in the bathroom to their favorite talk show as they're taking a shower, turn on the radio in the living room to their favorite

the candle exercise

To introduce yourself to concentration, create a practice for yourself as an extension of your sitting practice following posture and breathing. Once you have completed your breathing exercises, light a candle and place it on a table so that it is visible at eye level.

Return to your formal sitting posture with your hands atop your knees and your arms straightened for support. The practice is to maintain focus on the flame without describing it, analyzing it, or doing anything else that triggers a sequential thought process. Your mind will likely turn to pad thai, e-mails you need to send, or something else of interest to you, but simply return your thought to nothing but the candle's flame. You may find yourself thinking of a whole string of things completely unrelated to a candle for minutes at a time, but when you realize that this is what is happening, just bring your focus back to the flame without becoming frustrated or impatient. Your mind is, after all, of the same quality as every other person who has tried to bring stability and balance to their lives.

Start this exercise for a short amount of time, and then gradually build it up from there. The candle can be replaced with any simple object, such as a coin, a dot on the wall, a picture, or anything else that holds your attention. The practice, ultimately, is not to think about the object but rather to not think about anything else. For the amount of time you choose to practice this exercise, your task is to make that object your entire universe.

top-forty station as they're making themselves breakfast, and even leave all of these devices on simultaneously to make sure they have company wherever they go around the house. When work is over at the end of the day, they have two or three conversations with different people. They spend most of the day responding to e-mails and text messages and will likely repeat the same routine the following day. And the day after that.

Does this in any way resemble your life? Do you constantly fill your life with chatter and entertainment? With the many communication devices and other forms of stimulation available today, it's common for us to fill our lives up with activity and media. Often this need for stimulation stems from a fear of being alone or without decisive purpose. If we don't have anything to listen to in the morning, we might feel the need for someone or something to keep us company. If we sit on a city bus without something to read, we fear that we'll be bored. The irony, however, is that living a life without long periods of silent moments undermines our ability to enjoy the moments that we fill with music and talk.

To have a silent moment is to have a moment free of the need for stimulation. This can happen when working toward total concentration or meditation, but it doesn't have to be limited to the time spent on the mat following the practice of posture. Silent moments are actually the most beneficial in the time leading up to your craziest part of the day (for example, the first hours of your job after a long weekend, at the beginning of a day filled with many errands, or right before a noteworthy occasion like a wedding or important meeting). In fact, the best indication of your need for a silent moment is the very moment when you feel you have to rush to get things done, especially when you're about to make an important decision. Instead of giving in to that urge, take five minutes to be silent.

What are different ways that we can explore silent moments? We can try not putting on the radio or TV when we're getting ready for work in the morning. We can abstain from listening to music some of the time we're in our cars or on the bus. We can, quite simply, sit on our mats with our eyes closed for five minutes before we head off to take care of a laundry list of tasks. As you continue to explore your practice, work to find at least one silent moment—be it a morning without sounds or five minutes before a social event—each day. The most effective practice will be to find a moment of silence before the most hectic and crazy part of your day.

Finding more moments of silence in our lives will inevitably lead to greater silence in the mind. And, as we've already explored in many

practices for building awareness

different ways, a silent mind is a happy mind. For those of us with useful intentions, being silent and alone does not mean we are lonely.

understanding misinformation

Throughout the last hundred years, there have been many debates about the best and healthiest way to live. Some experts say that eggs are a healthy staple of our diets for their vitamins and protein while others argue that egg yolks' high cholesterol content poses a health risk. For many years it was felt that the best way to eat was to sample food from each of four food groups each day, but then in the early 1990s this construct was replaced with a pyramid favoring grains; the pyramid was designed by the branch of the government most interested in grain production and has been implicated in the increasing occurrence of type 2 diabetes in the United States. Even though water has been a staple of the diets of billions of organisms for millions of years, certain government agencies of the twentieth century declared a specific intake of water necessary for each and every person. Modern science has inspired an explosion of information. To what extent, though, can this information be trusted?

Receiving misinformation from authoritative sources is a defining aspect of modern culture. We are told how many calories to consume, how much water to drink, which vitamins we're supposed to take each day, and which amino acids can't be produced by the human body. However, diabetes rates have gone up, cancer rates have increased, obesity has skyrocketed, and many other mutations of our general health have taken place. We are receiving all of this misinformation because the people presenting it are either ignorant of the truth, or they have a commercial interest in certain information (that is, the industry creating the product wants to make money off your consumption of it, or news outlets want to sell you controversial stories about health in order to profit by them).

Looking to modern discoveries for health and lifestyle information is like trying to reinvent the wheel. Humans have existed for thousands of years by living within the natural order of all things, and the ancient yogis devoted years and years of meditation to gaining a systematic understanding of how we can use nature to define better health. These teachings refute many different modern strands of information about diet and nutrition, and here I isolate a few of these ideas as they were taught to me.

Calories: Calories are a unit invented by modern science to determine how much energy is contained in food. Modern nutritionists recommend that average adults should consume between 2,000 and 2,500 calories per day. It is misleading, however, to assign a general value of energy intake to everyone, as each of us has a different digestion process and different food needs based on our size and body type, and each of us participates in different forms and levels of physical activity. It is better to eat an amount of food that serves our own individual digestion needs, allowing that amount to shift during different seasons and to be defined by whether we need more or less energy.

Sugar: It is common and accurate to say that refined sugar and sweeteners like high-fructose corn syrup lead to weight gain and are detrimental to our health. In response, the health food market has developed many different ways to imitate the effects of refined sugars through substances like evaporated cane juice and brown rice syrup. Our bodies don't need sources of sugar that have gone through any of these types of processing, and the difficulty digesting such substances leads to weight gain and health problems. It is better to use honey, molasses, and maple syrup as the primary sources of sweetness in our diets.

Fat: A significant debate has taken place in recent years about how much fat we should consume each day, which fats are good for us and which are bad, and what percentage of calories in each food item we consume should be derived from fat. It is not useful, however, to assign a one-size-fits-all formula to fat consumption. When addressed through the Ayurvedic system, the questions of how much fat to eat and which fats to eat are based on which doshas are most dominant in our bodies at any given time and whether or not we consume cooler oils for warmer bodies and warmer oils for cooler bodies. A package may say that an energy bar has twenty grams of fat, but the package won't ever be able to tell you how much of the bar turns into fat when it enters your particular body.

Water: Modern science currently dictates that each of us should consume about two liters of water per day. Similar to fat intake, the amount of water we should consume is based on the amount of water we need to satisfy our thirst. Those who sweat more, such as people with excessive Pitta energy, will likely require more water than those with Kapha energy, who sweat less. Drink as much water as is needed to quench your thirst and no more.

Protein: The proponents of modern science, such as agents of the Center for Disease Control and Prevention as well as the U.S. Department of Agriculture, have told us that there are certain strands of amino acids that we are incapable of producing on our own. The absence of these strands in our bodies has formed the basis of the argument that we should eat large quantities of meats and other animal proteins. These types of food have low water content and are difficult to digest. The many millions of people who have sustained long, healthy lives over the many thousands of years of Ayurvedic practice are a testament to how unnecessary it is to consume such excessive quantities of animal proteins. We can get whatever protein we need from dairy, nuts, legumes, grains, and vegetables, and the prominence of these food types in our diets will enable the body to also produce protein itself. It is not accurate to say we need to consume protein when the body is quite capable of producing it from a natural and balanced diet.

In addition, those on the spiritual path of yoga do not take life, be it an animal's life or another human's life. This hinders spiritual progress toward higher states of awareness.

Vitamins and vitamin supplements: Artificial vitamins began being manufactured in the early twentieth century, and since then supplements have become a standard component of nutrition. Vitamins are defined as substances that the body can't produce on its own and must therefore be consumed or absorbed from external sources. Artificial vitamins are an altered version of the nutrients your body needs, but the body must work to stabilize itself in response to processing anything artificial or excessive. It is far more beneficial to eat a simple diet filled with fruits, vegetables, whole grains, and other natural foods to receive vitamins.

Detoxification: Even with an entirely natural diet of organic, locally grown food items, we will always have toxins in our bodies needing to be expelled. Between air pollution, noise pollution, and emotional stress, we build up toxic matter in our systems. Many members of the health food industry, such as self-help authors and sports nutrition vendors, have begun packaging overly complicated methods for enabling detoxification. Detoxification should be defined by what you take out of your body, the method you use, and determining whether or not the process harms the system in any way. The condition of the body must be taken into consideration, as the aftereffects may leave the body weak and open to disease. In the next section I provide a practice of fasting that helps to explain the Ayurvedic method of cleaning our bodies in a natural way.

fasting

If you go into any health food store or nutrition center, you'll find a section of products devoted to helping you cleanse yourself of the many toxins we encounter in the food, air, use of electronic gadgets, and stress of our daily lives. This can come in the form of special cleansing powders, supplements, specialty drinks, and the books and manuals to accompany these programs. They promise to reduce bloating, purify the colon or blood, and even convert carbohydrates into indigestible fiber to reduce starch intake. Sometimes these products are all bundled together into one nifty package and priced accordingly.

None of these products, however, are necessary for successful detoxification of the body.

Whether they're not in on the secret or they simply don't want you to know the truth, all of these companies looking to sell you something for detoxification are only providing you with distractions from what is ultimately necessary for cleaning yourself out. All you really need to do to successfully detoxify yourself is to consume nothing but hot water for several days.

Yes. Hot water. The human body is a part of nature and like the rest of nature has its own ability to clean itself out. We wind up getting burdened by the many toxins present in our everyday lives, and by further burdening ourselves with constant eating, we undermine the body's ability to detoxify itself. The body invests a lot of energy in digesting food, and when the job of digesting food is removed, the body is able to invest more energy in restoring balance. When a person is not digesting food, the feces loosen up and are able to move through the large intestine. Additionally, the hot water helps to break down and carry out the toxins as well as allows the body to rest from the intake of food.

Many yogis have used fasting to great effect, and there are many stories of fasting practitioners who lived particularly long, healthy, and conscious lives. One of the most famous examples of a person who fasted was Mohandas Gandhi. While most people associate Gandhi's fasts with a form of nonviolent protest, he also used them for self-purification. We can see the benefits of his purification through the depth of his capacity to live an entirely benevolent example for the sake of others. After all, he defeated the biggest empire in the world and freed India while never raising a finger. That is true power.

It is also worth noting that Gandhi's as well as most other stories of fasting took place before the invention of nutrition centers.

herbs

As I mentioned in the previous chapter, much of Ayurvedic medicine centers on the medicinal use of certain herbs. While modern medicine has made abundant use of artificially created substances in the form of

fasting

Beginning a fast requires no physical preparation, but it does require mental awareness. All that needs to be done at the beginning is to set an intention to fast at the beginning of a day before any food or drink has been consumed. Drink hot water throughout each day of the fast.

There are two potential benefits to a good fast. Before we begin, we must simply decide whether the fast is for mental or physical purposes. A physical fast happens when we want to remove toxic materials from our bodies. A mental fast follows the same pattern as a physical fast, but in practicing it we set an intention to clear our old and stale thoughts, habits, and lifestyles. Whether you intend to clean out toxic materials or toxic thoughts, having a detoxified system will allow you to invest more energy into your practice. A sign of a successful fast is when, after some days of detoxifying, the body and mind start to experience a lot of energy and lightness. This increase in energy will lead to an increased awareness, which in turn will lead to a heightened sense of consciousness.

Each of us will benefit from fasting for two days, but fasting any longer than that will depend on the type of body you have.

- If you have a skinny, wiry body like that of people with abundant Vata energy, then limit your fast to two or three days.

- If you have a medium build like that of people with abundant Pitta energy, then you can fast for three to five days.

- If you have a thicker, heavier build like that of people with abundant Kapha energy, then you can fast for four or more days.

I offer these guidelines to you, but without consultation, no one else can tell you how many days are best for you to fast. This should come from how your body and narcotics and other kinds of drugs, Ayurveda relies on natural herbs that the earth has created. The principle of favoring herbs over modern artificial pharmaceuticals is based on how the chemicals in pharmaceuticals take over the function of the body by entering the blood and overriding the immune system. In contrast, natural herbs only assist the body in its own defense against disease. The body becomes stronger each time it fights its own battles and weaker each time drugs undermine its ability to do so. In addition, using unnatural forms of medication requires the body to commit resources to processing them as foreign substances and to spend more energy detoxifying itself of them. The body accepts natural herbs as part of the essential food we consume as though we're consuming

mind are feeling during the process. If in the first few days you feel more tired, it can be because more toxins are being released and you will overcome this feeling. It can also be because you have not made a mental commitment and are resisting the process.

How to finish your fast depends on how long you have fasted, as abstention from eating diminishes the strength of the digestive fire. When your digestive fire isn't strong enough to digest the food, you will experience indigestion, stomachaches, gas, constipation, and malabsorption of food in the small intestine. If you fast for only two days, then you can begin eating the first morning after your fast with pureed, well-cooked foods like soups and natural (not icy) fruit shakes. If you choose to fast for three, four, or five days, then you should begin with liquids before eating solids. For the first morning after your longer fast, prepare a pot of basmati rice with about twice as much water as the recipe calls for. Once the rice is overcooked and mushy, the pot should contain several cups of water

holding nutrients from the grain. Drink a cup or so of this rice water as your first meal of the day, and then eat softer, pureed foods like the overcooked rice later in the day. By the second day after you've finished your fast, your digestive fire should be built up enough for basic solid foods like rice and cooked vegetables. By the third day, you should be able to resume your standard eating routine without any digestive complications. Remember that the longer you are on a fast, the more days you should take to reintroduce solid foods and return to normal eating.

You may fast up to once a week or more when needed. Please also note that fasting is not intended to be a means of losing a lot of weight in a short amount of time. The concepts of Ayurveda encourage the practitioner not to lose weight, but rather to attain a natural weight by living and following a natural, healthy routine and practicing natural habits. If you lose weight during the fast, you will inevitably regain most if not all of it when you resume your standard eating routine.

other plant life, like fruits and vegetables. Because of the potent, medicinal properties of herbs, however, we must be careful to use them in the ways and amounts that benefit the system.

A trained Ayurvedic therapist or herbalist is the only person who can and should prescribe herbs for certain conditions to be treated as based on this system unless a person reads and studies to know the qualities of herbal medicines. However, I've provided a sampling of herbs that you may already have in your kitchen cabinets that can be used on a daily basis for improving and supporting the body's health, vitality, and energy. Use these herbs as a part of your daily intake of nutrition instead of using vitamins and other artificial supplements. The first four you can make into a tea by using one-half to one teaspoon of the herb in a half cup of hot water. They can also be mixed together for increased potency. If you drink one to three cups a day, you will promote health and well-being as well as change the energy of your mind and body.

Turmeric: Turmeric is an herb native to India and other parts of South Asia. It is known for its orange-yellow color and use in curries. Using turmeric medicinally will reduce an overabundance of Kapha and Pitta energy. While it has a hot property, it does not aggravate Pitta energy. Turmeric can be used to control blood sugar level (diabetes), help skin disease, heal ulcers, purify the blood, help digestion, break up mucus in the respiratory system, purify the liver, and relieve congestion. Turmeric can be made into a paste and placed topically on the skin for swelling or bruises to decrease inflammation.

Ginger: Ginger is commonly used in the cuisine of many different cultures and has been cultivated across the world. Fresh ginger root reduces Vata and Kapha energies, and dry ginger reduces Kapha energy. Dry ginger has a much more potent effect than its fresh counterpart. Ginger can be used to relieve indigestion, strengthen digestion during meals, relieve respiratory problems, reduce coughs, reduce a running nose, help alleviate allergies, and help burn toxins in the intestines and stomach. Use ginger powder and a lemon juice to make a paste and apply it to the forehead to relieve headaches or a paste of ginger and water on joints to relieve pain.

Licorice: Licorice is known for the use of the plant's root as a flavoring in various candies and other food products. As an herb, licorice root's sweet and cooling properties can help reduce an overabundance of Vata, Pitta, and Kapha energies. Licorice is good for resolving respiratory issues, improving complexion, healing ulcers, soothing the voice, resolving hyperacidity, and calming the mind. It can also be used as a tonic for the heart and with milk as an expectorant. Only small quantities, such as half a teaspoon, are needed.

Tulsi: Tulsi is an herb that has been a staple of Ayurvedic medicine for thousands of years and is used as an elixir of life to promote longevity. It is known as a *tridoshic herb,* in that it can help balance Pitta, Kapha, and Vata energies, but its hot nature can aggravate Pitta energy if taken in excess. Tulsi helps resolve respiratory problems of cough and colds, helps clean the lungs, benefits the memory, helps resolve sinus congestion, helps resolve skin issues, and can improve the immune system. It also promotes higher energy in the brain and helps to clear the mind for spiritual practices. Tulsi can be found in Indian and health food stores in a tea or powder form.

Aloe vera: The aloe vera plant is commonly known in Western culture for its beneficial effects on the skin. Taking aloe vera as a supplement can help reduce Pitta energy and can balance all three of the doshas. Its cooling property can be used as a tonic for the entire body. It is very effective in resolving liver and spleen disorders, skin problems, (cooling) burns, hyperacidity, ulcers, colitis, and for constipation as a mild laxative. When used topically, aloe vera can be used to heal the skin and can cool and resolve the outbreak of herpes.

Once you use herbs as medicine in your daily life, you will feel these benefits as they have been explained to you.

ghee

When the Western world invented margarine, it became popular to shun the use of butter because of butter's large amount of saturated animal fat. When the Western world discovered the dangers of trans fats, butter once again became the more popular item. When the Western world created vegetable butter substitute products, well, the small plastic tub industry gained a large percentage of market share. Present for the last five thousand years and throughout all of these discoveries, however, has been ghee.

Ghee is known in the West as clarified butter and is a staple of Ayurvedic medicine and cuisine. Ghee is made by boiling off the water in butter, and when this is done the butter retains all of its healing properties without the moisture that instigates cardiovascular complaints and other issues stemming from the use of animal fat. Ghee is composed of short-chain fatty acids, which are known to be more easily digested into the blood than their long-chain counterparts found in butter. The body can therefore digest and use every part of ghee for nutrition, reducing the likelihood of it being stored as fat in the body. Ayurvedic practitioners have observed and noted the healing properties of ghee over the course of thousands of years.

What are the benefits of ghee? Consuming ghee helps to keep the body properly lubricated for the sake of healthy elimination. The muscles and bones benefit from the high absorption rate of ghee's nutrients, and the body's ability to easily digest ghee helps to kindle the digestive fire. Ghee can help with sexual debilities and even helps to remove harmful cholesterol. It is common to melt ghee over cooked vegetables and grains, though it isn't recommended to cook foods in the ghee itself unless done in low heat to preserve its goodness. It can also be consumed in the morning by placing a few tablespoons in half a cup of hot milk that has been boiled with raw cashews. A pinch of turmeric, cardamom, or nutmeg can also be added for taste. Consume this drink to help strengthen the body tissues, promote intestinal health, and calm the nerves.

Over time, the ancient sages learned that ghee can be applied not just through consumption as a food item, but in other medicinal contexts as well. Melt and put a drop or two of ghee in the eyes if they are red or irritated. You can also take a little bit on the finger and massage it into your nostrils to help clear congestion and nasal inflammation, to help induce sleep, and to avoid premature graying of the hair.

Ghee can keep without refrigeration for up to a year and can be found in Indian grocery stores and other venues associated with the Ayurvedic sciences. A life without ghee is no life at all!

sense control

Earlier we explored how excessive behaviors can stem from an ego-based need to gratify the senses and maintain control over getting what we want. We also noticed that constantly filling our lives with noise and chatter can disrupt our balance. Each of these ideas concerns our relationships to our senses and the impact of those relationships on our behaviors. If we smell some food and decide we must have it, we're indulging in our senses of smell. However, if we choose to control our senses instead of indulging them to excess, we create a greater opportunity for growth and peace.

The practice of controlling the senses is rooted in the traditions of yoga, as are posture, breathing, and concentration. This practice of controlling the senses centers on assessing which of our five senses is the most heightened and then curbing the amount of stimulation to that sense. When in college, we might go through a phase of indulging our senses of touch as we gratify our sexual urges through our newfound independence from our parents. If we feel particularly despondent about something that goes wrong in our lives, we may go through a phase of indulging our senses of taste through excessive eating. In these or any other phases, we have an opportunity to investigate our behaviors and create beneficial change.

What follows is a series of questions for each of the five senses. If we find that we're indulging one or more of these senses, it can become our practice to abstain from those behaviors through the processes outlined earlier in the book. I've also included an example of how to use one of the exercises presented earlier in relation to each sense.

HEARING

- Do I constantly listen to music while at home, in the car, on the bus, or while walking?

- Do I have to constantly be talking on the phone with someone or be in constant conversation with others? Do I do most of the talking when in those conversations?

- Do I have to always have one or more TVs on in the house even when I'm not really paying attention?

- Am I a better listener or talker?

If you listen to music during your commute, spend one week listening to music for only half of each direction of the commute. The following week listen to music for only half of one direction of the commute, and so on.

TOUCHING

- Do I engage in excessive sexual behaviors?

- Do I constantly require physical contact with others?

- Do I have to consistently feel the texture of items and objects I come into contact with?

- Do I have an aversion to people touching me?

If you have an aversion to people touching you, choose someone you trust, and schedule some brief hugs. For the first week, allow that person to hug you for a few seconds. The following week, allow them to hug you for half a minute, and so on.

SEEING

- Do I constantly watch TV or films?

- Do I need to always be in front of a computer even when not at work?

- Do I constantly need to watch everything that passes me on the streets or on the side of the road as I travel?

- Is my attention easily distracted by static or moving objects?

If you spend three hours a day watching TV, spend one week watching only two hours a day, the next week only one hour a day, and so on.

SMELLING

- Do I always need to indulge in food that I smell even when I had no intention of eating?

- Do I need to constantly use perfume, cologne, fresheners, and deodorants whenever I interact with others? Do I require someone close to me to use such substances as well?

- Does the smell of others or certain places turn me on or off?

If you use a certain amount of cologne or perfume each day, then spend one week using half as much, the following week using half as much again, and so on.

- Am I constantly eating?

- Do I need to always be drinking something like alcohol, coffee, soda, or other stimulants?

- Do I always need to have my mouth working by chewing gum, biting my nails, or smoking cigarettes?

If you smoke a pack of cigarettes a day, then spend one week smoking only fifteen cigarettes a day, the next week smoking only ten cigarettes a day, and so on.

Our senses are always working, and they benefit from resting during the day as well as when we're asleep. If you discover you are consistently indulging one of your five senses, then work toward relieving it of its burden. Once you have relieved the most heightened one, it's time to move on to the next one, and so on. One of the main parts of this practice is working toward having fewer desires and seeking less pleasure, and controlling the senses is a crucial aspect of this process. Here you will find balance.

self-study

At the beginning of the book I mentioned that it is common for people to pick up one spiritual book after another and make the simple act of reading books their practice instead of spending years trying the exercises provided in them. One might buy a book, read each page of it, and when finished put it down and exclaim, "Brilliant, I know this stuff!" then immediately pick up another one and repeat the same process. This is an act of seeking inspiration but not direction.

However, it doesn't mean that once we've found a practice we must stop reading spiritual books. If you choose to pursue the practice outlined in this book, there are many texts that can teach you more about the joy and peace that form the basis of your path. These texts can include ancient Indian scriptures like the Yoga Sutras and the Bhagavad Gita, or they may include other ancient spiritual texts like the Bible, Tao Te Ching, or Torah. But if we choose to pick up another book that is not an ancient text, how do we know if we are simply trying to find inspiration without direction?

Self-study begins by asking ourselves why we are reading what we are reading. Self-study requires us to explore the difference between picking up a book for the sake of increasing our sense of personal truth and picking it up to avoid the practice outlined in the last book we read.

Take a look at your bookshelf. Are there dozens of other books that outline a practice like the one outlined in this book? Did you read those books but never try their exercises? Is this book about to become the latest addition to that shelf? The act of self-study might begin with receiving instructions from a book or teacher, but what we do with those instructions determines the quality of our practice. If you practice the exercises outlined in this book for six months or a year, you will likely find that you are ready to refine your practice of those exercises, and you may be tempted to search out more books to gain this information. Do not worry about where to find guidance. Instead, put your energy into practicing daily, and as you evolve through this practice, the next level will come to you naturally. The next time you find you're looking for more reading material, I encourage you to consider the following question: Have I been studying and practicing what I already know daily for many years, or do I have a habit of spiritually jumping about?

cultivating sexual energy

Many of us have sex on our minds for much of the time we're alive. We think about whether we're getting enough of it or wonder when we'll get it again. If there's any doubt about how much our society thinks about sex, all we have to do is look at how many advertisements are filled with women in bikinis or turn on a sitcom making jokes about male member size or attend a stand-up comedy show featuring cracks about involuntary celibacy. Sex plays a large role in our cultural lexicon.

From a yogic perspective, there's a simple reason for the significance of sex in our day-to-day lives: sexual energy is one of the most powerful energies we have. Much of the energy and essence of food produced by our bodies is committed to ensuring our ability to produce sexual energy. This makes perfect sense, as the activities of procreating and sustaining life are so important.

The problem, however, is that most people indulge in excessive sexual practices by spending their sexual energy many times each week. Because the body must work so hard to produce this energy, constantly regenerating it drains other vital life forces. Those who have too much sex will tend to be fatigued and experience dullness in their eyes and minds.

By contrast, abstaining from excessive sex provides an opportunity to channel this abundant form of energy into other ways of living, be it practicing a physical discipline, using it to bring greater focus to our work, building better relationships with others, or exploring a creative outlet. The practice of cultivating and guarding our sexual energy centers on finding a balance between having a satisfying release of sexual energy, channeling part of the energy in creative ways, and not allowing the energy to spill over in sexual frustration, as it may with people who experience too little sex.

You can explore your own practice of sexual activity to see if you are using this life force in a way that ensures the greatest possibility of sustained health and balance. To determine whether or not you practice excessive sex, assess your general sense of energy and vitality. If you feel you spend much of the day experiencing fatigue, then try reducing the frequency and amount of sexual release and observe what happens. If, with reduced sexual activity, you feel a renewed sense of vigor, then you may benefit from a diminished sexual routine. If you feel that withholding release causes frustration and irritability, then you may benefit from channeling the energy in either a sexual or nonsexual way. Also, be sure to avoid excessive sex during the hotter, more humid months of the year so as to avoid dissipating the body's energy through dryness.

choosing the higher path

I once heard a story of a woman who suffered the loss of her daughter at the hands of a man who raped and then murdered the child. Rather than rally for his execution or simply hate him with as much ferocity as her grief could inspire, she visited him in prison on a regular basis. Over time, she worked to help him rehabilitate himself, and together they forged an unlikely friendship. She was asked why she chose to befriend and support the man who had ended her daughter's life. In response, she said that if she had avenged her loss, her daughter would have suffered through a horrifying death, she would have suffered through the pain of her loss, and her daughter's murderer would have suffered as he rotted away in prison. By reaching out to this man, both of them found a higher purpose for themselves, and the number of people who suffered was reduced to one.

There are many times that we feel wronged by others, and the easiest and seemingly most satisfying response is to antagonize them, reject them, and even retaliate with some sort of vengeful act. However, as we saw when discussing nonviolence, perpetuating such negative emotions in response to others only furthers our suffering and certainly won't serve anyone else. When we have a conflict with another person, we have an opportunity to create a stronger, healthier bond with that person by reconciling our differences, as did the woman with the prisoner. This will create greater peace within ourselves. I encourage you to explore this practice in any way you can, no matter how difficult.

sacrifice

A young student went to his guru to receive help in finding his practice.

"How do I find joy?" the student asked the guru.

"Eat less food," replied the guru.

"Eat less food?" said the student. "But I'm not fat."

"Eating less will give you more time for other things," replied the guru.

"I enjoy my food an awful lot. I don't know that I could make that sacrifice."

"If eating less helps you to feel better," said the guru, "are you really making any sacrifice at all?"

The student considered this.

"I suppose," said the student, "that attaining greater health wouldn't really be a sacrifice."

"Perhaps," said the guru. "And if you continued to eat as you do, what sacrifice might be made then?"

The student considered this.

"If I ate more food than I needed," he said, "I suppose I'd be sacrificing my health."

"Perhaps," said the guru.

. . .

Sacrifice is a word that seems real only when we are at the beginning of the journey. Once we are on our way we realize that there was no such thing as sacrifice, there was only an opportunity to live in a more beneficial way.

fill in the blank

The following chapter provides an outline of how to incorporate all of the practices in this book into one cohesive practice. Before moving ahead and reading this final chapter, pick at least one practice from chapter 9 and add it to your daily routine for several days. This will help you to further ground yourself in the demands for a personal practice when devising your own routine in response to chapter 10.

union

putting it all into 10 practice

WHEN I FIRST STARTED studying in India, I was living in Madrid. I spent two months in India and then returned home to Madrid to attend to other matters. While in Spain, I was diligent in maintaining the practice I had cultivated in India with the help of my guru: wake up at 5:00 a.m.; drink some hot water; practice posture, breathing, and concentration; have breakfast; drink herbal concoctions; attend to the matters of my day; and sit once again before going to bed at 10:00 p.m. I felt light, focused, and ready for just about anything.

Except, perhaps, for the arrival of Pino.

Pino and I had been friends for a number of years. He worked as a concert promoter for some of the biggest acts in the world, including U2 and the Rolling Stones. Because the biggest concerts in Spain were in the country's two biggest cities, he kept a home in Barcelona and liked to crash at my place when in Madrid.

"After all, Cameron, your neighborhood has the best restaurants in the city," Pino would tell me. Pino loved going to restaurants. And clubs. And bars. And parties. And, of course, concerts.

Three days after I returned from India, Pino showed up at my door. It was 9:00 p.m.

"Cameron," he said, "it's been ages."

"How are you, mate?" We hugged.

"Hungry. I haven't eaten in over an hour." He dropped his bags by the door and headed to the kitchen.

"You're in Madrid for a few days, then?" I called after him.

"U2 is in town for a few shows. You know, the usu—*Cameron!*"

"What's wrong?" I ran into the kitchen.

"There's no food in your refrigerator!" He was standing with the door of the fridge wide open. In it was an assortment of fruits and vegetables, some milk, and half a loaf of bread.

I tried not to smile at the stricken look on his face.

"Well, I don't really keep leftovers or anything. I've been keeping things simple since I got back from India."

"From India?" he asked. "What are you, some kind of yoga man now?"

I shrugged.

"Is that where you got this?" he asked, picking up a canister of ghee from the counter.

"Oh, yes," I said, "that's ghee, or clarified butter. It's a staple of Ayurvedic medicine and cuisine."

Pino looked at me for a moment and then left the kitchen to return to the front entrance.

"Well?" he said.

"Well what?" I replied.

"I'm not going to wait for long. Let's get your pants on, then."

"Why do I need pants?" I asked, looking down at the pajama trousers I had bought in India.

"To go out to eat, of course." He continued to wait by the door.

"Sorry, mate, I don't eat this late anymore. I'm going to be in bed by ten."

"That's fine, I just want you to come down for a quick bite, anyway. You can be back here by ten."

I knew my friend, knew of his persistence, and loved him for it. After the pants were on, we went down the street to his favorite Italian restaurant.

When we returned to the flat at midnight, we had had appetizers, shared several entrees, had dessert, and gone through two bottles of wine—well, he had, anyway. Our "quick bite" wound up being more food than I had eaten in the last two days put together. When I woke up the next morning, I was so tired I skipped over my practice so that I could sleep later. It was four days until I reclaimed my preferred routine once again.

Eventually Pino went home, and I went on with my life as well. After visiting family in England and New York, I returned to India and spent another two months there. At the end of those two months, I returned to Madrid and continued with my practice. I woke up at 5:00 a.m.; drank some hot water; practiced posture, breathing, and concentration; had breakfast; drank herbal concoctions; attended to the matters of my day; and sat once again before going to bed at 10:00 p.m. I felt light, focused, and ready for just about anything. I maintained this routine for two weeks without any distractions.

"Cameron, it's been ages," Pino said as he walked through my door two weeks and one day after I returned from India. We hugged.

"How are you, mate?" I asked.

"Hungry. Busy. You know, the usual."

"I'm not going to be able to go out tonight," I said. "I've got to be in bed by ten."

"I know. You're Señor Yoga Man now. That's fine. I have to work tonight anyway."

"Oh, yeah?" I asked, relieved that he wasn't going to try to wine and dine me. "What's the show?"

"Oh, no, Yoga Man, you're not interested in concerts anymore."

"Well, no," I said, "I was just asking you about your work."

"Sure," he said, "but you don't care about Lenny or any of my work. You just care about vegetables and ghee."

"Lenny?" I asked.

"Oh, *sí*. Lenny Kravitz is performing at Plaza de Toros de Las Ventas."

Las Ventas was one of the biggest bullrings in the world.

"But, like I said, you're not interested in concerts." He went to attack my empty fridge.

Lenny Kravitz was perhaps the only recording artist whose concert could entice me away from the vegetables. My friend knew me well.

After the concert I made to part ways with Pino and his friends.

"No, you can't go, Cameron, you've got to stay for the after-party."

After being at the after-party for an hour, I told Pino that I needed to head home. It was one in the morning.

"Stay a little longer, Cameron. How often do we get to see each other?"

At three in the morning, one of Pino's friends puked in the bathroom. I helped Pino bring him out to a cab to send him home.

"I think I've got to go home too," I told my friend as the cab drove away.

"Lenny and his crew just got here," Pino said. "Things are just starting to get going."

From the party people's perspective, I must have seemed like a rather docile presence in that I drank only herbal tea, didn't get into anything crazy, and was one of the first to leave at seven in the morning. Several others had passed out on the floor of the club and seemed rather content not to go anywhere. From the perspective of my practice, however, I not only didn't go to bed at ten, but I didn't even get home until after I would have otherwise been up for several hours for the start of the new day.

. . .

The next thing I'm supposed to write is "After staying out until 7:00 a.m. and spending an entire evening with people whose sole purpose was to become intoxicated to the point of passing out on the floor, I never allowed this lifestyle I didn't want to lure me away from my practice again." I'm supposed to write this, but I can't. I may have set a significant intention to change my life upon Ron's death, but I had almost no willpower to sustain my practice when presented with distractions.

This makes perfect sense. Building a practice is not an easy thing to do, as the nature of our minds urges us to indulge the senses and seek as much of what we call pleasure as we possibly can. Of course I used to prefer to eat a lavish meal and have an occasional drink instead of going to bed at 10:00 p.m. Of course I'd prefer to see a Lenny Kravitz concert in a bullring than get up early the next morning and practice postures for an hour. While many centuries of yogic tradition and many different contemporary practitioners demonstrate that developing a spiritual practice leads to peace and joy, we are often so entrenched in the material world that it is inconceivable that living another way is even possible—let alone joyful or beneficial.

This chapter is written to respond to exactly this challenge. It is fine for me to offer practices related to nonviolence, full breaths, and sticking clarified butter up the nose, but how does a person move toward this from their typical habits of yelling at the TV, taking shallow breaths, and slathering their large, greasy muffins with butter? Creating your practice will be a lifelong journey, and it's unreasonable to think that you'll be able to practice every exercise in this book every day from the moment you close the book until the moment you pass away many years from now. That doesn't mean, though, that there's anything stopping you from taking your first step.

the ideal schedule

Because they are thousands of years old, the systems of yoga and Ayurveda predate modern inventions like business lunches and rush-hour commutes. Here in the twenty-first century, we face the challenge not only of developing the discipline to practice new and different ways of improving our lives, but also of doing so in the context of many social and professional obstacles. The ancient sages may have been thorough in passing information to their students down through the centuries, but they didn't think to teach them how to squeeze in a posture practice when their friends are trying to drag them to a Lenny Kravitz concert.

If we were to eliminate all modern distractions from our day-to-day lives and be dropped off somewhere in the Himalayan mountains, we would have no problem following the daily schedule outlined below, which is actually my daily routine as defined by the systems of Ayurveda and yoga. These guidelines are set out to give the practitioner perfect balance between mind and body as well as bring the personal balance of Pitta, Kapha, and Vata into equilibrium if one or more of them is out of balance with nature.

SET AN INTENTION

If you haven't already done so, go back to chapter 2 and review the guidelines for how to set a proper intention for your practice. Though this is something that you won't do every day, it is very important to do it at the beginning and to revisit it every couple of months. Be sure to incorporate your contemplation and other related practices into this part of the process.

MORNING

Rise before sunrise: The energy when the sun rises is very powerful and makes the body feel alive. The sun is the heat energy of the world and helps everything to awaken and warm up. We benefit from being in sync with this powerful rhythm and even shifting our morning routines to change with the earlier or later sunrises of each season. Many of our health issues will disappear just by adjusting our inner clocks to the outer balance of nature and this powerful force.

Start the day by drinking a cup of warm water: This will help the digestive juices of the stomach to gain strength and will help to eliminate waste from the body.

Look at the tongue and eyes: Is the tongue coated with a white or yellow film? If so, there are toxins in the stomach or colon. Are the eyes excreting any liquid? This can be from the creation of excess mucus and from eating and drinking late the night before. If the eyes are red or dry, then the habits from the day and night before weren't healthy and need to be adjusted.

Sniff a little warm water mixed with a pinch of salt up each nostril: This will aid in the release of excess mucus buildup during the night and open up the nasal passages. This process will alleviate any problems of asthma or allergies. The nasal passages also need to be clear for clarity of thought.

Practice posture, breathing, and sitting quietly for some time: Incorporate the practices outlined in chapters 6 through 9 into your daily routine for greater balance and for developing tools to deal with life issues as a whole. Begin with the twelve-posture sequence in chapter 6, but also begin to work with the Kapha, Pitta, and Vata sequences as they relate to your imbalances.

Decide whether or not to take a shower: Bathing too much dries out the skin, so unless you get dirty on a daily basis, it is not necessary to shower every day. What is more, we do not usually sweat as much in the winter, so taking a shower each day during the colder months isn't necessary either. On a daily basis we can use a cloth to wash the face, under the arms, in the groin and buttocks, and the feet.

Put oil on the head: Rubbing some Ayurvedic oils or sesame, coconut, or almond oil on the head and massaging it into the scalp helps the mind to calm, improves the general health of the scalp, and helps avoid the drying or graying of the hair.

Have breakfast: Most people consume sweet desserts for breakfast, such as pancakes, waffles, French toast, muffins, white toast with jam, pastries, cereals, doughnuts, and other baked goods. None of these foods have much nutritional value or are beneficial to the system. They also aggravate the system and will contribute to a person becoming overweight and excessively dry.

If you have excess Pitta energy, having a little breakfast is fine but not of heavy, sour, or spicy foods. Instead, have a moderate amount of simple foods that tend to be naturally sweet. This can include but is not limited to fruits, grains like rice, and light dairy products like milk and feta cheese. Take a tablespoon of aloe vera a few times a day, and drink other cooling herbs such as cumin, fennel, or coriander as a tea infusion to relieve any Pitta-based stomach or digestion issues.

If you have excess Kapha energy, then an early breakfast is not beneficial for you. Eating later in the morning after 10:00 a.m. is better. Foods should be light, like fruits, soups, and vegetables. Avoid sweet things with the exception of having a little honey with other foods.

If you have excess Vata energy, an early breakfast is beneficial for you. Breakfast should be lubricating to the system. Ghee, olive oil, and butter should be consumed. Avoid dry foods like toast, crackers, and cereals. Dairy is good.

Start work: We have an opportunity to bring the calmness we experience in our practice into the attitude we bring to work or another daytime environment. We share the energy we created with our practice with others through greater patience, understanding, and kindness. No matter how your co-workers, children, or others act, do not react with anger or hostility. Allow others to be the way they choose. This adds to our spiritual growth.

AFTERNOON

Eat lunch: Lunch is not a necessity for excessive Kapha imbalances, but if eaten it should be a smaller amount and take the place of dinner. However, just because it is lunchtime doesn't mean that you need food and should eat. Lunch can be moderate in size for excessive Pitta imbalances, but if you're feeling heavy, then missing lunch is better. Lunch helps to root the body for excessive Vata imbalances.

Silence: Either during a lunch break or in another environment, spend some time sitting in silence as suggested in the "Sit Before You Veg" exercise in chapter 1 or the silence practices outlined in chapter 9. Taking even five minutes for yourself will help you to stay focused during the rest of the day, and you will benefit from doing this many times before going to sleep that night.

EVENING

Silence: Practice the "Sit Before You Veg" exercise from chapter 1 before eating dinner. Incorporate this silence into the dinner itself by eating without distractions like television or reading. You will feel less hungry and more aware of your surroundings and the people in it. Stress will make you eat more!

Eat dinner: Dinner should be no later than 5:00 p.m. for excessive Kapha imbalances and should be the lightest meal of the day. Foods with more water content like vegetables or fruits are best. Excessive Pitta imbalances can again be offered a moderate amount, but it should be the smallest meal of the day. For Vata imbalances, dinner can be a little later, at around 7:00 p.m., and food can be in the same quantities as before. Also consider missing dinner entirely, as doing so is a healthy practice.

Drink an herbal tea: Make yourself an herbal tea, as suggested in chapter 9. Allow this tea to follow your final meal of the day to better aid digestion.

Practice one exercise from chapters 3–5: Practice one of the various exercises based on chapters 3–5, such as observing the news commentator (chapter 3) or writing a letter (chapter 4). If you have an excessive Pitta imbalance, favor exercises based on the nonviolence practices in chapter 3 to help abate frustration and anger. If you have an excessive Kapha imbalance, favor the detachment exercises in chapter 4 to help remove indulgence and heaviness. If you have an excessive Vata imbalance, favor the excess exercises in chapter 5 to foster greater contentment with stillness and quiet. Commit fifteen to thirty minutes to an exercise each evening. This practice will help in you letting go of nonbeneficial habits you keep coming back to later at night.

Place oil in the nose: Rubbing a little ghee, sesame oil, or coconut oil inside the nose before sleeping helps the mind to calm at bedtime, keeps the nasal passages clear and lubricated, and helps to aid breathing. This can also be done after washing the nose out with salt in the morning.

Go to sleep: To foster greater balance, it is best to allow the body the rest it needs and not to keep it up late. Staying up late will increase the chances of experiencing insomnia and creating greater nervous energy throughout the next day, which then leads to a mountain of other health problems. Sleep is hardest if you have an excessive Vata imbalance, and so bedtime for people with excessive amounts of this energy needs to be a little earlier than the other dosha imbalances. The best time would be around 9:00 p.m. for Vata, 9:30 to 10:00 p.m. for Pitta imbalances, and 10:00 p.m. for Kapha imbalances. Avoid sleeping on the stomach, which is not good for breathing.

Allow natural urges: Never stop or block the passage of the natural urges of sneezing, burping, passing gas, yawning, sexual release, urination, defecation, or coughing.

Don't use antiperspirants under the arm, as blocking these sweat glands will cause rashes to appear on the skin and create issues in other parts of the body.

Enjoy sunlight: Make sure the face and body get a few minutes of sun each day, as this is food for the skin.

Avoid too much talking: Be an observer without an urge to be verbally overexpressive or to constantly offer your opinions to others.

modifying the ideal schedule

Okay. If you've gotten this far into the chapter, that means you're still interested in change. You may have noticed that this ideal schedule requires several hours of your time every day. If you're like most people, you might read this list of tasks, throw your arms up in the air, and say, "Yogi Cameron is crazy! There's no way I can find the time to do all this stuff!" Given how much of a struggle it was for me to stick to my practice when my friend Pino came into town, I can certainly relate to your frustration. After six years I worked up to a daily practice like this that lasts three hours. This is my lifestyle as well as my vocation, and it's a practice that needs to keep growing if I am to better assist others in their practice or in treating them. While this practice may be an ideal way to live, it is likely a dramatic departure from your current lifestyle and is not necessary for you at the beginning, just as it wasn't for me. The key is to do the practice and not just think of doing the practice, which is why it is often useful to start out with a sampling of this routine at first and then grow it over time.

I would therefore like to present a modified, scaled-down version of the above routine. I have created three different versions of the practice for you to explore, as defined by the three different energy imbalances of the doshas. I have arranged these routines in this way because balancing our bodies is a helpful first step in balancing the rest of our lives. With bodies in greater balance, we often find that we can make time for all sorts of things and create many opportunities for ourselves and others. Below are three lists of tasks to begin your practice as based on each of the three doshic imbalances. Refer back to the dosha quiz in chapter 8 to remind yourself which energies are most excessive for you right now.

THE PITTA ROUTINE

If you're experiencing excessive amounts of Pitta (fire) energy, you will likely be completely gung ho to begin this practice and try everything all at once. What will probably happen, though, is that you will take the practice too far to the point of burning yourself out. This can then lead to frustration, self-hate, and anger. To help settle this energy, begin your practice with the following five tasks:

- Make a tea of cooling herbs like cumin, fennel, coriander, and turmeric. Drink this tea several times throughout the day.

- Practice gentle forms of posture with an emphasis on breathing at the end.

- Avoid too much stimulation in the form of direct sunlight in the middle of the day, excessive chatting, and eating when overly emotional.

- Practice a nonviolence exercise from chapter 3 each evening.

- Practice the silent lunch exercise with a friend once a week.

THE KAPHA ROUTINE

If you have more of a Kapha (earth) imbalance, you'll take a long time to get into a routine like this and then possibly get stuck in one part of the practice without the ability to grow into it further. To help you to move the heaviness of this energy, try the following tasks:

- Wake up before 6:00 a.m. during Vata time to create movement.

- Practice posture, particularly the Kapha sequence in chapter 8, and other physical activities to move the heavier earth energy.

- Avoid mucus-producing foods like heavy dairy products, meat, and sweet foods.

- Eat dinner before 5:00 p.m. to avoid eating in the Kapha time of day and the heaviness that accompanies such a habit.

- Avoid drinking too much liquid (water, juices, soft drinks, alcohol), especially during meals.

- Practice a detachment exercise from chapter 4.

THE VATA ROUTINE

If you're experiencing imbalance as a result of excessive Vata (air) energy, you're likely to jump into this routine with every intention to change your life. You're also likely, however, to become distracted from it within a short period of time and then flit in and out of the routine in the ensuing weeks or months. To help this energy to calm down, practice the following tasks:

- Find several moments to sit in silence both at the beginning and the end of the day.

- Practice posture for lengthier periods of time, and spend time sitting in stillness at the end.

- Incorporate a concentration practice into the morning routine, such as the candle exercise in chapter 9.

- Incorporate essential oils into the diet, and apply oils to the body, per the above routine and the information found in chapter 9.

- Use the excess exercises from chapter 5 to help temper the sexual release of energy on a day-to-day basis.

- Go to bed by 9:00 p.m., during Kapha time, to help bring rooting energy for deeper sleep.

The intention behind practicing this more simplified routine is to help you get used to creating a practice of greater awareness and balance throughout your life. It is likely that more than one dosha is out of balance, so you should begin incorporating practices from more than one of these routines for better balance.

It is important to remember to take what we can from this type of routine but also to keep adding more and more to our daily lives. Ultimately, the goal is to attain and experience such an improved sense of balance in our lives that in the future we have the time and patience to do everything in the original routine.

knowing ourselves a little better every day

It is my intention that you will use this book as a way to introduce yourself to greater awareness in your life. I hope you set proper intentions to begin freeing yourself of the material world and that you create the change that this type of path has promised and delivered to the many millions of people who have walked it over thousands of years.

Ultimately, everything in this book has been presented to you with the intention of teaching you how to find the most natural and free version of yourself. This is not a short journey or a particularly easy one. However, nothing stands in the way of your greater self becoming a complete and total reality. This is a practice of spending at least part of each day learning a little bit more about yourself than you did the day before, and the more you learn about yourself, the more content you will be. Ultimately, it becomes a practice of being guided by the guru in you.

. . .

About a year after our colorful times with the Lenny Kravitz crowd, Pino and I were enjoying a leisurely late morning in the living room of my apartment while he was in town for another concert. I had been up for several hours. Pino had been up for several minutes after a particularly late night and was disgruntled by his inability to lure me out with him. My willpower had grown.

"Here's what I don't get about you, Cameron," Pino said from the couch. "You say you don't want to indulge in these 'excessive forms of living,' as you call them. But look how extreme you are in the opposite way. Don't you think you need to live?"

"I am living, Pino. Very much so."

"You spend an hour sitting still and drink *ghee* for breakfast. What kind of life is that? You need balance. The old Persian poets were all about wine, women, and song. Live now, as who knows what can happen tomorrow?"

"But how do you think the poets felt," I asked, "when there weren't any women and wine around?"

Pino shrugged and then collapsed into the couch and closed his eyes. He seemed more tired than usual these days, as though his lifestyle was starting to catch up with him.

"During my training," I said, "I heard a story from the Hindu scriptures about two men who encountered a great sage named Narada on his way to Lord Shiva's place—"

"I don't want to hear any of your voodoo stories about people with ten arms, Yoga Man." He reopened his eyes, but only just.

"Okay, fine." I thought for a moment. "Then I'd like to tell you a different story."

"Mmmm . . ." Pino closed his eyes again.

"Right. So, there were two concert promoters—"

"Ooo!" Pino said, opening his eyes wide. "Was one of them a devilishly handsome man?"

"Only on the outside," I said.

"What?"

"Oh, never mind. Anyway, both men worked very hard at their jobs and wanted to do well. The first promoter pitched his clients to five venues every week, and the second promoter did the same. One day a prominent entertainment journalist came through the city where both men lived.

"'Where are you going?' the first promoter asked the journalist when he saw him walking by. 'To the president of a major media conglomerate,' the journalist replied. 'I'm looking to report on the major acts present in this city this weekend so that the conglomerate can consider sponsoring them.' The promoter knew that sponsorship from a company like that would be a huge boost to his career. 'Could you let me know what he's looking for so that I can increase the chances of my clients getting sponsored?' The journalist replied that he would, and continued on his way until he encountered the second promoter.

"'Where are you going?' the second promoter asked the journalist. 'To the president of a major media conglomerate,' the journalist replied. The journalist then told the second promoter about the sponsorship opportunity. 'Could you let me know what he's looking for,' the promoter asked, 'so that I can increase the chances of my clients getting sponsored?' The journalist replied that he would.

"The following day the journalist was once again journeying through the city when the first promoter saw him again. 'Mr. Journalist Man!' he said. 'Did the president tell you what he was looking for?' 'He did,' the journalist replied, 'and he said that he only wants to work with names that are on the rise, so to be considered for the sponsorship you must pitch your clients to ten venues every week.' 'Ten venues!' the promoter yelled. 'But I already make my pitch to five venues! I would have no time for wine, women, and song!' 'If that is how you feel,' the journalist said, 'then the opportunity is probably not for you.'

"The second promoter then saw the journalist and likewise asked him what the president said. 'He told me that he only wants to work with people who take their work seriously,' the journalist said. 'He said that he will consider you if you pitch your clients to twenty venues every week.' 'Oh, is that all?' the second promoter replied, not knowing it was twice as many venues as was assigned to the first promoter. 'I thought he was going to ask me to work more hours than there are in a day. At least I know how much more work I need to do. I'll get started on that right away.'

"'Actually,' the journalist said, 'you don't have to do that at all.' 'What do you mean?' asked the second promoter. 'That you've accepted such a task as making your pitch to so many venues, I know that I can depend on you to do the work that needs to be done to be successful. The sponsorship is yours.' 'How can you speak for the president of a major conglomerate if you're a journalist?' asked the second promoter. 'Because,' said the journalist, 'the president is me.'"

I looked at my friend, who had been listening to the story to the end.

"So," Pino said, "what you're saying is that I have to work four times as much to find happiness?" He raised his eyebrows. I could tell that he was playing dumb for theatrical effect.

"Yes, you could do that," I said, "but the story is meant to show that the one who accepts his path as timeless with no expectations of getting certain results will find greater happiness in life. Both promoters were asked to do more work even though they were already working very hard. While the first promoter balked at doing anything more, the second promoter accepted it and detached from getting any results. If we do the work with the intention to grow and be beneficial to others rather than use the work as a means for getting the next buzz in life, we'll live in contentment rather than suffering."

"Because eating vegetables and sitting for an hour will help us to know ourselves."

"It's a beginning but, yes, eventually."

"And always looking for the next pleasurable thing outside of ourselves will continue to disappoint us."

"Right."

Pino brooded over this for a moment. I figured it wasn't necessary to tell him that the president was based on the great sage I had mentioned earlier, and the sponsorship money represented ascension into a higher state of being.

"Well," he said, getting up from the couch with a groan, "it's a cute story, Yoga Man. Let's get your pants on."

"For what?" I asked, still sitting.

"The pub's about to open. It's time for a drink." He smiled as he went to the kitchen. I heard the refrigerator door open and waited for the usual moan.

"Maybe," I said, mostly to myself. No matter how much breathing I did, how many times I sat in silence, and how much I pursued this path, there was always going to be a Pino ready to distract me from the work. In the end, all I had to do was remember my intention to keep coming back to the practice.

Pants would be optional.

. . .

Visit yogicameron.com to learn more about apps for furthering your practice.

acknowledgments

My first acknowledgment goes to the creator, with the hope for each of us to be aware of this energy and guided from within.

To Amy Hughes and David McCormick at McCormick & Williams, thank you for all of your help in bringing this book into being.

To my editor Eric Brandt, my gratitude and love for the confidence you placed in this book from day one and all of your support of the process. You have been inspiring to work with. To Cynthia Ditiberio, many thanks for becoming such an enthusiastic supporter of this book and for taking the many steps required to see this editorial process through to the end.

My thanks go to Suzanne Wickham, Kathryn Renz, Carolyn Holland, Priscilla Stuckey, and all of the good people at HarperOne for making this book a reality.

Thank you to Dr. Vasudevan, my teacher, for guiding me along the Ayurvedic path these past years. You have added to my path in a very significant and loving manner.

To Neil Gordon, thank you for all the help with writing and the creative process we went through together all these months. Much love to you.

To Jaimyse Haft, my gratitude and appreciation for all of your hard work and interest in spreading the significance of the yogic path. To Shab Azma, thank you for all your support and help in taking little and turning it into creative work.

Thank you to Maria Menounos for your staunch advocacy of the Ayurvedic way and for all of your excellent work in supporting its message.

To Dr. Hari for supporting my practice with attention as my teacher.

Thank you to Kali and Rudra from Integral Yoga for teaching me the art of yoga sadhana from my first teacher-training course.

Thank you to the talented Holly Millea for being a wonderful friend, something each person needs in life.

Much gratitude to my parents, Iraj and Theresa Alborzian, who have been examples of love by accepting my choices without prejudice or judgment.

My deepest thanks go to Almudena, mi mejor amiga in life who has shown me love and kindness all these years.

And, finally, much warmth and peace goes to my daughter and love Azusena, who is an example of a beautiful human being and my greatest inspiration.

acknowledgments

the questionnaire of marjorie, the pitta energy example

First name: Marjorie

Age: 25

Sex: Female

Health Issues: I experienced a recent benign tumor of the salivary gland and had it removed. I am currently healing.

Does your body feel more hot or cold? Hot.

How large is your body frame (S-M-L)? Small to medium.

History of past illness (if any): I had a colonoscopy at age 15 for bloody stools and hemorrhoids.

Dietary habits: Do you eat a vegetarian diet? I do for the most part, but I do sometimes eat fish and also eat dairy.

Time of meals: Breakfast: 8:00–10:00 a.m.

Yogi Cameron responds: Make sure to first have a cup of warm water before eating anything. Make breakfast very light or just liquids, such as vegetable juice or fruit juice (not acidic or sour fruits). This will build up the digestive power for a meal.

Lunch: 1:00–2:00 p.m.

YC: Have your first meal starting around 10:00 or 11:00 a.m., which will support digestion. Foods can be heavier than those eaten at dinnertime.

Eat the dairy, rice, legumes, and other denser foods here so they have a longer time to digest.

Dinner: 7:00–8:30 p.m.

YC: This can be a little earlier, at around 5:00 or 6:00 p.m., to give more time for digestion to happen before bedtime. Make this the lightest meal of the day with foods like vegetables (not root vegetables) and soups (not tomato), and avoid too many hot spices. Also, be sure to add two to four spoonfuls of ghee to your food at mealtimes.

Appetite: What quantity of food do you eat in one sitting? Medium to large quantities.

Name five foods that you commonly eat each day/week: Bananas, cheese, eggs, spinach, tomatoes

YC: All foods but the spinach are not benefiting your health at this moment. They are heavy and will hinder digestion, which is one of the main issues to alleviate at the moment.

What tastes are you more attracted to? Salty foods.

YC: Avoiding salty, sour, and pungent foods for a while will bring the fire/Pitta issue into balance.

Do you eat leftover, frozen, microwaved, canned, or precooked foods? I eat leftover, frozen, canned, and fried foods.

YC: These are all heavy, nonbeneficial foods that can ruin the digestive process.

What types of drinks do you consume? Water, tea, orange juice, wine.

YC: Avoid wine, tea, and acidic beverages like orange juice for now. Drink water only when thirsty, and start to add some herbal teas into your daily routine. Try some ginger, cumin, and fennel teas. There are other Ayurvedic formulas as well, but start with these for now as they are available to you right away. Avoid cold iced drinks.

What types of snacks do you eat? Salsa, chips, and guacamole.

YC: Salsa is too spicy for your system.

How often do you snack each day? I don't usually snack, or sometimes once a day.

Where do you eat most of the time (home/restaurant/work)? I eat at both home and work.

What digestive issues do you have (pain, gas, constipation, etc.)? I can sometimes have gas and also get constipation.

YC: This will all clear up with the new eating routine.

Do you get bloated? Yes.

YC: This is the result of the food not being completely absorbed.

Do you drink and eat at the same time? Yes.

YC: In excess this will lead to indigestion, bloating and constipation.

Do you eat in a quiet environment? I try to do so.

YC: Try harder (just joking).

Do you eat in silence or while being social? I usually eat while talking.

YC: This will cut off the breath each time you converse and hinder breathing as well as digestion.

Lifestyle choices: Do you smoke? No.

Do you drink alcohol? Yes.

What medications or pills do you take (how many and for what)? I take an anxiety medication two to three times per week and wear a birth control ring three weeks out of the month.

YC: These medications have a toxic effect on the body. They make the hormones in the system imbalanced, and many side effects arise from both prescriptions. The anxiety comes from excessive thinking and focusing on one thing for too long. This does not bring us peace. Once this has shifted, then there is no use for antianxiety pills. It is better to also find alternatives for birth control, such as condoms, because chemical substances throw the system out of balance and make the nervous system function erratically. Through treatments and practice, you can come off these very easily.

Do you take drugs? I sometimes smoke marijuana.

Do you take supplements (vitamins, etc.)? Yes, I take vitamins, probiotics, fish oil, evening primrose oil, and vitamin C.

YC: This is a lot for the system to digest at once.

Have you tried diets/detoxing? Yes.

Do you tan artificially or naturally? Yes.

YC: Avoid artificial tanning, as it ages the skin and doesn't benefit your health.

Do you spend a lot of time thinking about things? Yes.

What kinds of thoughts repeat themselves? I often think about my family, my self-worth, guilt about not doing enough, goals I have set for myself, my happiness, my health.

YC: An excess of Pitta often brings on these emotions, as too much fire energy makes a person competitive.

Generally, do you talk a lot? Yes.

YC: All the above lifestyle choices are related, as one will feed the other. For our minds to be peaceful, we must speak little, listen a lot, and pick the moment to think and say something of worth to the world. Otherwise, our lives are a whole lot of wasted moments and talk.

Sleep habits: What time do you go to sleep? Midnight.

YC: This is contributing to your nervousness. Move this to 9:30 p.m., and you will see a big difference with your behavior and emotions.

What time do you get up in the morning? 7:00 a.m.

YC: This is okay, though a little earlier may be better.

How many hours do you sleep each day? Six to eight.

Do you sleep during the day? No.

YC: In the summer heat a short nap at the hottest point of the day will benefit you.

What is your usual position when you sleep? I sleep on my back.

YC: Good.

How do you feel in the mornings? I usually feel pretty fresh, though sometimes it's hard to get up on weekdays.

How would you describe your sleep? Deep.

YC: Great.

Do you wake in the night? I sometimes wake up, but not often.

Exercise habits: What types of exercise do you do? I run, cycle, swim, play basketball and tennis, and do Pilates and yoga.

YC: As per our conversation, these are all very active and energetic exercises, and we need to bring a little calmness in between them to balance out this fire. Some yoga postures, breathing, as well as some concentration practices will benefit you.

How often do you exercise? I typically exercise four to five times per week.

Do you sweat a lot? Yes.

YC: Your sweating needs to lessen and will balance itself out once you reduce the heart rate and activities.

Do you get short of breath quickly? No.

Do you get cramping in the muscles? No.

YC: This is a sign of good muscle health.

Work environment: What is your profession? I produce films.

How many hours do you work each day? It depends, but I usually work between eight and twelve hours a day, and either five or six days a week.

Do you work at night or during the day? I work during the day.

Do your eating habits change, such as when you go overseas? No.

YC: Incorporate seasonal foods into your diet when traveling.

Do you work in an air-conditioned environment? No.

YC: Good.

What sort of nervous issues do you have? I do tend to get nervous when stressed out. I take the nervous pills for a reason!

YC: Through the yogic practices the mind will slow down and thoughts will become controllable. It is dedication that is needed and not a certain amount of time committed to practicing. A part of your new practice is to focus on self-growth.

Home environment: How many people live in your home? I live with two other people.

Do you live in a noisy house? It depends on the day. While I wouldn't call it a noisy house, I can't say it's quiet all the time, either.

How many hours per day do you watch TV? I watch one hour per day.

YC: Good.

What types of TV do you watch? I'll usually watch comedies or dramas, but I don't watch that much.

How many hours a day do you use the computer, cell phone, or other electronic devices? I use a computer and cell phone all day for work, and then for about one hour outside of work.

YC: Try to break from this for a moment each hour so the nervous issue is not fed on a constant basis. Too many electronics make the nervous system overstimulated with foreign invisible rays. Not healthy.

Do you use air-conditioning? No.

YC: Good.

What are your hobbies? I like to do photography, cooking, exercising, and painting.

Travel habits: How often do you travel and how long is the journey? I usually only fly between LA and NYC, so it's typically a six-hour flight. I make this trip about ten times a year. I travel for personal reasons about three to four times per year.

YC: When flying, wear a mask to avoid air pollutants and viruses. Also put some oil in the nose and take some herbal teas like gotu kola with you to calm the mind. Stand and stretch during the flight as much as possible.

What modes of transportation do you take? I use planes and trains.

What climate changes do you endure, if any? It varies, but I mainly experience the climates in NYC, the Midwest, and LA.

YC: When traveling, be sure to adapt to the seasonal foods in that area instead of eating the same things you would eat at home.

Sexual habits: Do you find your sex life satisfactory? I generally find it to be above satisfactory, but I've made a few comments on that below.

How often do you have sex? I usually have sex daily, but that depends on whether or not I need to travel for work.

YC: This is too much and will tax the system as well as dull the mind. Try to find other creative outlets, or put some of this energy into your hobbies.

Do you mostly engage in sex during the day or at night? It mostly happens at night but sometimes happens in the morning as well.

YC: Later at night after 10:00 p.m. is not a good time for exchange of this energy for people of too much Pitta/fire energy.

What other issues or comments do you have regarding sex? Sex is mostly enjoyable for me, but I haven't been having orgasms lately. The act itself is sometimes dry.

YC: Sex is more of a mental act than a physical one. When the mind is busy and moving a lot, you will not be feeling in the mood as often. Given how busy and distracted you can be, it is difficult for you to have what might be considered a normal sexual urge. Also, when the body is not healthy, a person is not as sexually active. Try this earlier in the morning during earth time, and see if it makes a difference, as you may be more relaxed and thinking less.

Stool pattern: How often do you move your bowels? I tend to go one to two times a day.

YC: This is good.

What is the texture of your stool? It's usually pretty solid, and sometimes a little bloody.

YC: This can be caused by too much fire in the system. This may also be from small hemorrhoids or the skin at the exit of the anus. As it is light and little in quantity, it does not suggest anything severe.

Does your stool sink or float? It floats.

YC: This is healthy.

Is your stool dark or light? It depends, but it's usually light.

YC: If it is always light it can be because of your diet, but if you eat a large variety of foods and it is still light then it can be a liver issue.

Does your stool have a strong odor? It varies.

Urine: How frequently do you urinate? I urinate frequently, and get sudden urges.

YC: The amount you sweat and the extensive physical activity you participate in should lead to less frequent urination. Your frequent urination and getting sudden urges may be coming from consuming diuretics like black tea, sweet drinks like orange juice, and caffeinated beverages.

Do you ever urinate during the night (awakening from sleep)? Yes.

YC: It's best not to drink anything up to an hour before bed so your sleep is not interrupted.

Does your urine have a strong smell? It depends.

What is the color of your urine? It is usually clear but can be dark yellow after I take vitamins in the morning.

YC: The body is excreting these vitamins, making them excessive. Be sure not to take too many, and taking none at all would be even better.

For women: Menstruation: Do you experience any menstrual pain? No.

YC: Great.

How many days does your period last? It lasts four to five days.

YC: This is healthy.

Is there much bleeding during your period? No, there is only a little.

Is your blood dark or light? It is more on the lighter side.

What activities do you engage in during your period? I still engage in work and sports.

YC: Try to avoid sports as it is not a good thing to do during your period. Rest and contemplation are ideal for spiritual growth.

Do you experience blood clots during your period? No.

YC: Good.

How would you describe your relationships:

. . . with your friends? I have very loyal friends and we're happy together. I'm often surrounded by humor and insightfulness.

. . . with your partner (if applicable)? It's a thoughtful and committed relationship. He also brings much humor and passion to our experiences together. He's definitely my best friend.

. . . with your parents? They are very supportive and greatly important in my life. I'm very similar to my mother, yet we can sometimes butt heads. I get along with my father very well. They are two very emotional relationships.

YC: With a daily practice, you will learn to detach from some of these emotions. Observation is a good tool for this. Watch and have little opinion of what others say, and you will be able to just see them as they are. The advantage here is that you will be able to better ground yourself and not get carried away by your emotions. No one will be able to bother you from this point of view.

. . . with co-workers? I have strong friendships with my co-workers, almost as if we're a family. They are accepting of me, and the relationships continue to evolve.

. . . with yourself? For the most part, I really like myself. I do put a lot of pressure on myself to succeed and to reach new levels.

YC: Your practice will also help you to find a balance between inner success and outer wants. Be patient, but become aware of your thoughts on a daily basis to see if any one or more thoughts have power over your emotions. You will find calm and balance through breathing techniques.

the questionnaire of jennifer,
the kapha energy example

First name: Jennifer

Age: 33

Sex: Female

Health issues: I have fibroid tumors.

YC: As fasting and herbal medicines have been used for thousands of years to heal many ailments, doing this may be the correct method for breaking down the tumors and evacuating them from the system.

Does your body feel more hot or cold? Hot.

How large is your body frame (S-M-L)? At 5'9" and 210 pounds, I'd say I'm medium to large.

History of past illness (if any): None!

Dietary habits: Do you eat a vegetarian diet? No, but I grew up vegetarian as a child.

Time of meals: Breakfast: N/A, as I'm never hungry in the morning. I'm a late eater (after 8:00 p.m.), but really I just eat anytime I want.

YC: Not eating in the early morning is beneficial for you, but late eating has the reverse effect, as that will help put more heavy earth element onto the body.

Lunch: 1:00–1:30 p.m.

YC: This we could also make later in the afternoon, and then cut out dinner. Otherwise, the dinner will likely add weight to the body.

Dinner: I usually grab fast food or eat out after 6:00 p.m.

YC: Fast food may be fast, but it has little nutrition. After eating fast food, the body will crave more food, as it does not get the nutrition it needs. The nonbeneficial fat will also be stored and difficult to lose.

Appetite: What quantity of food do you eat in one sitting? Medium. My fibroid tumors take up abdomen space, and therefore I'm not hungry a lot.

Name five foods that you commonly eat each day/week: Pinkberry, cookies, candy (and anything else sweet), salads, anything with meat . . . I don't grocery shop.

YC: Most of these are the worst foods you could feed yourself. Sweets turn to more fat, as does a lot of meat. This is the recipe for a high blood sugar level and high cholesterol.

What tastes are you more attracted to? Sweet and salty foods.

YC: Astringent, bitter, and pungent tastes are more beneficial to your earth imbalance.

Do you eat leftover, frozen, microwaved, canned, or precooked foods? Yes, I eat leftover and fried foods.

YC: Both of these lesser foods are heavy and depress the system.

What types of drinks do you consume? I drink water and sometimes drink alcohol.

YC: Drink water only when thirsty, but also minimize it during eating. Sip warm water during meals to aid the digestive process. Your digestion is slow and is in need of strengthening. You need to be much more aware of protecting it.

What types of snacks do you eat? Cookies, candy, chips, and fast food.

YC: This is not food.

How often do you snack each day? Ugh . . . frequently. I eat a lot of snacks at work.

Where do you eat most of the time (home/restaurant/work)? I usually eat out at restaurants or grab food on the go.

YC: This again is hindering the digestion in the stomach and intestines, and helping to pass undigested food into the blood. It is toxic to the system.

What digestive issues do you have (pain, gas, constipation, etc.)? I get constipated and bloated when I eat dairy.

YC: You have a lot of excess fat and mucus in your body, and dairy will add to all of this, aggravating the excessive earth element issue even more. This will also happen with meat, sweets, ice cream, and any other deficient foods that are processed. Think natural.

Do you get bloated? With dairy, as mentioned above.

Do you drink and eat at the same time: Yes.

YC: Ginger tea with a pinch of pepper is best during meals and during the day. Only drink about half a cup during meals to avoid diluting the acid of the stomach and hindering the digestive process.

Do you eat in a quiet environment? No, I'm always on the phone, watching TV, or in a noisy place.

YC: You are not consciously feeding the body but just dumping food inside to fill up. The body is storing a lot of fat for this reason.

Do you eat in silence or while being social? Usually I eat while talking.

YC: This is hindering digestion as well as creating an imbalance in the mind. One who talks a lot has a head full of ideas but will rarely take action.

Lifestyle choices: Do you smoke? Yes.

Do you drink alcohol? Yes.

YC: This will add to your weight but also place a lot of pressure on the kidneys and liver. The blood will also suffer from toxicity.

What medications or pills do you take (how many and for what)? I take one iron pill a day for anemia.

YC: With the nonbeneficial foods you are consuming, there is no chance of this being digested or used in the body. It becomes another hindrance to the body and eventually the mind.

Do you take drugs? No.

YC: Good.

Do you take supplements (vitamins, etc.)? I just take the iron pills.

Have you tried diets/detoxing? Yes.

YC: The methods and herbs you use to detox need to be consumed in quantities in line with your body and not according to the package. The quality of the herbs (hot or cold) is also important as they may disturb the balance of the system.

Do you tan artificially or naturally? No.

YC: This is good, as tanning is very bad for the skin. It is of no benefit to the system and is dangerous.

Do you spend a lot of time thinking about things? Yes.

YC: This is where the yoga breathing will bring balance and calm to the mind.

What kinds of thoughts repeat themselves? I usually have negative thoughts about not feeling worthy, that I'm not able to do something right, or that I'm not good enough.

YC: Here we change the thoughts through yogic breathing and concentration practices to shift away from nonbeneficial movements of the mind.

Generally, do you speak a lot? I'm in the middle. I'm not a yapper, but I'm not quiet once you get to know me.

Sleep habits: What time do you go to sleep? Midnight–1:00 a.m.

YC: This is really disturbing the mind and making the body dry, nervous, and depressed. It brings about uncertainty of the mind, ideas, and thoughts. It makes a person more emotional.

What time do you get up in the morning? 8:00–8:30 a.m.

YC: It is best to wake up before sunrise to start helping the mind to become alert and alleviate the heaviness of the body.

How many hours do you sleep each day? I sleep about six to eight each night and still feel tired.

YC: The amount of sleep may be sufficient or may be too much, but either way your diet is requiring your body to constantly digest during sleep. This doesn't give the body an opportunity to rest.

Do you sleep during the day? Yes, I love naps.

YC: This makes and adds to the heaviness of the body and mind. Avoid this for now.

What is your usual position when you sleep? I sleep in a fetal position.

How do you feel in the mornings? I feel drowsy and tired.

YC: This is a result of your eating pattern and staying up late.

How would you describe your sleep? I usually have interrupted sleep.

Do you wake in the night? Yes.

YC: This is all a result of your various eating and sleeping habits. Here we will set up new habits and lifestyle changes.

Exercise habits: What types of exercise do you do? I don't do any exercising at all.

YC: Practicing some energetic yoga postures three times a week will change the whole shape of the body. You need movement to start changing the energy of the body, which will affect the mind in a positive manner.

How often do you exercise? N/A

YC: This needs to change for greater health of the body and mind.

Do you sweat a lot? N/A

YC: Some sweating is necessary for the health of the skin and the body.

Do you get short of breath quickly? Yes.

YC: This is a sign of not breathing correctly or not receiving enough essential gases to be able to function naturally.

Do you get cramping in the muscles? Yes.

YC: If persistent, it will affect the tone and strength of the muscle. You may also be short of essential salt, sweat and urination balance in the system.

Work environment: What is your profession? I am a strategy consultant at a not-for-profit agency.

How many hours do you work each day? Seven.

YC: As you are working only seven hours a day, there is much time for you to devote to changing many of the aspects of your daily routine.

Do you work at night or during the day? During the day.

YC: As I have suggested for you to not eat at night, it may be best to volunteer or take up a hobby to get you out of the house and keep you occupied. Find something you are passionate about.

Do your eating habits change, such as when you go overseas? No.

Do you work in an air-conditioned environment? Yes.

YC: This is stopping you from sweating some of the necessary toxins out.

What sort of nervous issues do you have? I get nervous when I drink coffee.

YC: It is best to avoid coffee, as the body is showing you.

Home environment: How many people live in your home? It's just me.

YC: Good. You have no distractions from others to stop you on your new path of healthy changes.

Do you live in a noisy house? No.

YC: Great.

How many hours per day do you watch TV? I watch from when I get home (7:00 p.m.) to when I go to bed (midnight–1 a.m.).

YC: This is creating a lot of lethargy and adding to the weight gain. Going for walks and being outdoors will help open the body after sitting in the stale environment of the office.

What types of TV do you watch? I favor mindless programs on MTV and BET as well as comedy shows and movies.

YC: As you recognize the nature of these programs, it is better to watch other, more positive programming or taking up reading of spiritual material. This will help you on your new path.

What types of music do you listen to? I love everything, including classical, rap, alternative, and world music.

YC: Try to avoid using headphones too much as the close proximity of the music to the eardrum will throw off the balance of the body. (Ears are a center of balance in the body.)

How many hours a day do you use the computer, cell phone, or other electronic devices? I use the computer about thirteen hours a day. Between texting, talking, and e-mail, I use the cell phone throughout the day for about two to three hours total.

YC: Extended use of the computer adds a lot of strain to the eyes, which can bring on migraines and eye strain.

Do you use air-conditioning? Yes.

YC: As above, avoid air-conditioning as it will hinder your ability to burn toxins and excess fat.

What are your hobbies? I don't have any.

YC: The mind is not stimulated or passionate about having a purpose in life. Here lies some of the feeling and emotions you are experiencing.

Travel habits: How often do you travel and how long is the journey? I haven't traveled in the past two years.

YC: Travel is great education and stimulation for the mind. The mind can be stimulated simply by going on hikes or for walks.

What modes of transportation do you take? When I do travel, I travel by plane.

What climate changes do you endure, if any? None.

YC: This is why it is important to stick to seasonal foods so the body is not consuming foods from very cold climates.

Sexual habits: Do you find your sex life satisfactory? No.

How often do you have sex? None.

Do you mostly engage in sex during the day or at night? I mostly have sex at night when I do get it.

What other issues or comments do you have regarding sex? My fibroid tumors make sex painful.

YC: This energy is being conserved, which is positive, but it needs to be expanded on some interests or artistic/creative ideas so there is a fulfillment in your life. You may become very frustrated if this energy does not find an outlet. Here, through yogic practices, you will learn to control and expand it.

Stool pattern: How often do you move your bowels? I have bowel movements every day.

YC: Good, as you should evacuate as many times as you eat meals.

What is the texture of your stool? It is solid.

Does your stool sink or float? It usually sinks.

YC: This isn't healthy, as it's a sign of undigested or heavy foods.

Is your stool dark or light? It is dark.

YC: This will depend on what you eat.

Does your stool have a strong odor? No.

YC: Good.

Urine: How frequently do you urinate? I urinate twice a day.

YC: This is a low amount for your body size, as you are retaining more water. This is not healthy unless it is the dead of winter and you are not drinking many liquids. Otherwise, the air-conditioning is inhibiting the sweating, which is the other way of excreting toxins as a liquid.

Do you ever urinate during the night (awakening from sleep)? Yes.

YC: Avoid drinking close to bedtime.

Does your urine have a strong smell? No.

What is the color of your urine? It is usually dark yellow.

YC: You are retaining a lot of water, as you also do not sweat very much. This can become troublesome to the tissues, creating puffiness or inflammation.

For women: Menstruation: Do you experience any menstrual pain? I only have slight pain.

YC: This is great.

How many days does your period last? It lasts exactly seven.

YC: This is a little excessive and will come down once you become healthier.

Is there much bleeding during your period? There is heavy bleeding on the second day, but it's light the rest of the days.

YC: Good. After the first or second day, bleeding usually becomes lighter.

Is your blood dark or light? It is dark.

What activities do you engage in during your period? None, I just rest.

YC: Great. This is a good, healthy action.

Do you experience blood clots during your period? Yes.

YC: If they last many days, this can turn into a health problem.

How would you describe your relationships:

. . . with your friends? My relationships are fine with the few friends I have.

YC: You attract the number and kind of friends that you want. Observe them, as they are quite similar to you in energy.

. . . with your partner (if applicable)? N/A

. . . with your children (if applicable)? N/A

. . . with your parents? We get on each other's nerves every now and then, but we get over it eventually. It's normal, I guess.

YC: It may be normal, but you can still observe them to see what your similarities are, and with this information you can work to change the negative traits. I know this is easier said than done, but this can be practiced through yoga methods.

. . . with co-workers? I just started a new job, and they seem okay.

. . . with yourself? I don't really have one, as it seems like work gets in the way.

YC: This is one of the first things to change. Having an understanding of oneself is the beginning of the path of self-realization or self-understanding.

Other personal comments: Oh, my god . . . this has really opened my eyes. I need some kind of balance. Please help.

Also, I grew up on Eastern religion and have known Paramahansa Yogananda's ideals on life and living all my life. As far as meditation techniques, I've used some Kriya yoga tools. I grew up vegetarian, meditating, and doing energization exercises and yoga before it was cool but have yet to get my life together.

YC: If this is part of your background, it will be helpful to start looking back and picking up some of these again as you will be familiar with them. The mind will hold onto something, and that is why we start having a spiritual practice. Each and every day, the mind will hold onto the reality and not a fantasy. It is important that we start to get you a spiritual practice so balance comes back into your daily routine. One must also know one's purpose in this life for contentment to rule the heart.

the questionnaire of christina,
the vata energy example

First name: Christina

Age: 38

Sex: Female

Health issues: Chronic constipation, sciatica, and entrapment of the hamstring muscle, hypothyroidism

History of present illness (if any): I have had sciatica and hamstring entrapment since 2003. My gynecologist recently discovered a lump in my breast. I plan to see a breast specialist later this year.

I have experienced significant hair loss in the last few months.

YC: The lump could be anything and typically can be taken care of if you go on a fast for about a week. There are many of these fat deposits that come and go, but the body will digest any cysts or tumors that come about due to stress or internal toxins not being flushed out. If you find it necessary, follow up with an oncologist or another Western medical professional upon completing the fast to monitor the progress of your condition.

History of past illness (if any): I have had hypothyroidism and chronic constipation since childhood. I was anorexic from 11 to 15 years old. I suffered from bulimia from 16 to 30 years old.

YC: Because of the last two illnesses, the air (Vata) element in your body has not been traveling downward to help the cleaning of toxins, aid in food digestion, and help in the elimination process. This air has been moving up, disrupting all natural urges such as passing gas, having the correct period flow, and a healthy sexual urge. This has caused an imbalance with all doshas but especially in the air element.

Dietary habits: Do you eat a vegetarian diet? Yes, and I make primarily vegan food choices without eating eggs or dairy.

YC: It would be best to incorporate dairy into your diet for now to get more moisture in your body. Eat foods in season. Don't mix too many foods together at the same meal for easier digestion. You also need essential oils in your system, which you are not getting.

Time of meals: Breakfast: I eat fruit and either tea or coffee at 9:00 to 9:30 a.m.

YC: Cut out coffee for now as it dries the kidneys and puts pressure on them. Move this meal a little earlier so it will be eaten during earth time and be heavier in your system. This will help you ground more.

Lunch: I have steamed veggies with brown rice or chopped veggie salad with vinegar and oil at 1:30–2:00 p.m.

YC: Try white (basmati) rice because it is easier to digest. Overcook it a little, and drink the rice water with the meal when you make it at home.

Dinner: I tend to have salad or raw veggies with hummus, or a puree of veggie soup with flaxseed at around 8–8:30 p.m.

YC: Hummus is made of beans and therefore can be a little heavy to be eaten at night. Instead, eat that at lunchtime. Keep your food quantity down, as it should not be overloading your system or make you feel very full, or else the digestion will suffer. Stay off raw foods for a while until the digestion is back to normal. Raw foods need much more digestive power. Your last meal should be around 7 or 7:30 p.m.

Appetite: What quantity of food do you eat in one sitting? Small quantities.

Name five foods that you commonly eat each day/week:
Vegetables

YC: Make sure to eat seasonal vegetables and to cook them.
Fruit

YC: These should not be acidic or too sweet like pineapples.
Hummus

YC: Cut this down a little as the digestion is not strong enough to process it in great amounts.
Gluten-free crackers

YC: These are very dry and will give more issues with constipation.
Fiber bars

YC: These bars are too concentrated, dry, and processed. It is best to eat natural foods, which have water and oil content as well as natural food nutrition.

Do you eat leftover, frozen, microwaved, canned, or precooked foods? No.
YC: Good!

What types of drinks do you consume? Water, coffee, teas, lemonade, almond milk, coconut water.

YC: Cut out tea as it contains too many stimulants. Lemonade is not good either, unless it is made from lemons, milled, and not too concentrated. Stay away from cold drinks, as they will aggravate your condition even more. Drink warm or hot drinks. You need calming and nurturing things and people for now.

What types of snacks do you eat?

Raw veggies with hummus.

YC: This is difficult for you to digest. When eating heavier foods, it is better for you to have white rice (basmati), cooked veggies, legumes (well cooked), seeds, and perhaps a few nuts but very few.

Gluten-free crackers or rice crackers and trail mix.

YC: These are way too dry for your system and will add to more constipation. Better fruit and natural products.

How often do you snack each day? I snack one or two times a day.

Where do you eat most of the time (home/restaurant/work)? I eat at work.

YC: When eating, only eat with your mind on the food. Don't eat during work, while on the computer, while using your cell, etc., as unconscious eating makes the mind think it has not gotten enough food. It is also very bad for digestion.

What digestive issues do you have (pain, gas, constipation, etc.)? I have severe constipation.

YC: This issue will clear up as you start the new approach to eating and the diet mentioned above. Also don't worry about too much variety for now as your body is so dry in the bottom half that we need to get you first going to the bathroom every day and then adding other food in.

Do you get bloated? Yes.

Do you drink and eat at the same time? I rarely do this.

YC: Start to drink some warm water or hot water with fennel powder during the meal. Alternatively, you can sip it after you have eaten.

Do you eat in a quiet environment? Most of the time.

YC: This is a good practice.

Do you eat in silence or while being social? I do both.

YC: When talking during eating, the body will become dry, the stomach bloated, and the mind restless.

Lifestyle choices: Do you smoke? No.

YC: Good choice.

Do you drink alcohol? Occasionally.

YC: For now, stay away from alcohol as it will dry out the body more and make the constipation and bloating worse.

What medications or pills do you take (how many and for what)? None.

YC: This is good.

Do you take drugs? No.

Do you take supplements (vitamins, etc.)? Yes.

YC: Consuming these requires a lot of digestive power and can make the digestion weaker. Having a balanced diet will deliver natural vitamins to the system.

Have you tried diets/detoxing? Yes, I've done the master cleanse.

YC: The ingredients for this cleanse make for a spicy, acidic mix that is often used to lose weight, so it will be counterproductive and very destructive to your already dry and overheated system.

Do you tan artificially or naturally? Yes, I tan naturally when away on holidays.

YC: Be sure not to burn or overheat the system.

Do you spend a lot of time thinking about things? Yes, I spend too much time thinking about things.

YC: Start to watch your thoughts, but don't stay in them. Through yogic breathing and concentration practices, you will think a lot less.

What kinds of thoughts repeat themselves? I tend to have positive, joyful thoughts of me being in total happiness.

YC: This is a very positive and beneficial practice.

Generally, do you speak a lot? Yes.

YC: This will dry out the vocal cords and give you an empty feeling, as if you need more air. It will make you tired and depressed.

What are your favorite topics of conversation? Travel, different cultures, the art gallery world.

Sleep habits: What time do you go to sleep? Midnight or 1:00 a.m.

YC: This needs to be at 9:00 to 10:00 p.m. and no later. By going to sleep at the heavier Kapha time, you will bring your elements back into balance. This will help quiet the mind. For you, going to sleep late at night will disturb the mind's balance and the body's rhythm with the sunrise and sunset.

How many hours do you sleep each day? Five.

YC: It is better for your nervous condition to sleep a few hours longer. After you have made a yogic practice for yourself each day, then sleeping less will benefit you, but for now you need more grounding.

Do you sleep during the day? No.

YC: If you are living in very hot temperatures it will be beneficial to maybe rest in the heat of the day so the body does not become more dry.

What is your usual position when you sleep? I sleep on my left side or my
stomach. I don't use pillows.

YC: Stay off the stomach and the left side. Sleep on the right side
(masculine-male-sun), as the body is abundant with the opposite type
of energy. We need to bring it back into balance.

How do you feel in the mornings? Tired and stiff.

YC: This will change with new habit changes.

How would you describe your sleep? Interrupted and light.

Do you wake in the night? Yes.

YC: These sleep habits are all going to come into balance once we get you
into a more natural rhythm, as described before.

Exercise habits: What types of exercise do you do? I run 25–30 miles a week
and do kickboxing, weight lifting, and Pilates.

YC: Hatha yoga will be better for your nerves and the balance between
body and mind. During these vigorous exercise practices, the breath
is very irregular and is affecting your whole life energy. It is making
your system very tired. I will show you new yogic breathing and posture practices, which will balance the air element in your system and
restore strength to your muscles.

How often do you exercise? I exercise five to six times a week.

YC: This is a lot for the fragile state of your body.

Do you sweat a lot? No.

YC: The body is telling you that the exercise is very excessive. You are
running a lot but not sweating, as there is little moisture for you to sweat
out. The body has become very dry from exercising in this fashion.
More nurturing rather than rapid and heating practices are needed.

Do you get short of breath quickly? Yes.

YC: This is significant, as noted above.

Do you get cramping in the muscles? Sometimes.

YC: The body is responding to excessive habits and behaviors.

Work environment: What is your profession? I work as a travel journalist.

How many hours do you work each day? 10–12 hours.

YC: As you are working much of the time you are awake, it is imperative
to stick to a healthy schedule of habits.

Do you work at night or during the day? Both.

Do your eating habits change, such as when you go overseas? Yes, sometimes
I incorporate dairy into my diet when I travel to Europe.

YC: As you travel a lot, it is essential that you keep the body lubricated with oil, both ingested and applied externally. Given your excessive Vata energy, the foods can be fattier than usual.

Do you work in an air-conditioned environment? Yes.

YC: It is important for you to get out of the building and walk when possible, as the air-conditioning will make the body even drier.

What sort of nervous issues do you have? I don't have any nervous issues.

YC: We all have nervous issues at times, and it up to us to recognize them and breathe through them. We will practice this when we meet. Here it is important to recognize oneself and the traits we have constructed.

Home environment: How many people live in your home? It's just me.

YC: I know this is something you do not like about your situation, but it does give you more time to practice many of the habit changes I have outlined. When you become healthier in the mind, you will also attract someone on this path as well.

Do you live in a noisy house? No.

YC: Great.

How many hours per day do you watch TV? I watch about a few hours a week, but not much.

YC: Good.

What types of TV do you watch? I watch the Food Network, the Travel Network, and VH1 Classic.

What types of music do you listen to? I listen to everything except country and hard-core rap or rock.

YC: It is good for your mind to stay away from loud music, which will disturb peace of mind. Quiet, calming music will be more beneficial.

How many hours a day do you use the computer, cell phone, or other electronic devices? 8–10 hours per day.

YC: This is not a healthy practice.

Do you use air-conditioning? I only use air-conditioning at work, as it is controlled by the building.

YC: Open the windows or take walks outside when possible.

What are your hobbies? I enjoy traveling to new countries to explore cultures, and I also like to cook and bake.

Travel habits: How often do you travel and how long is the journey? I travel very frequently for my job, and some journeys take as much as ten hours each way.

YC: This amount of movement in the body on such a regular basis is very negative for the nervous system as well as the body as a whole. It will make the body and mind susceptible to illness, so be sure to spend a lot of your time outdoors when you are in different cities. Over time, all of the artificial air, light, and foods will take their toll on the system.

What modes of transportation do you take? I travel by planes, trains, and automobiles.

What climate changes do you endure, if any? The climate frequently changes from warm to cold to dry to wet, depending on where I'm traveling to.

YC: Be sure to eat seasonal foods in each country, and avoid mixing different food groups in the same meals, as your digestion might suffer.

Sexual habits: Do you find your sex life satisfactory? No.

How often do you have sex? Right now, I don't have any sex.

YC: This will preserve your energy and give you more clarity of mind as you do your yoga practice.

Do you mostly engage in sex during the day or at night? Neither right now.

What other issues or comments do you have regarding sex? The only issue is that I am not having any sex as I am single and don't really like to sleep around. Just one man is enough, but there is no one man right now!

YC: As you are still thinking about the previous relationship, you cannot move forward and be with anyone else at present. The last relationship you had was not balanced in the sense of two people coming together to share, but it was one looking after another until they did not feel useful any longer. To not have to experience this again it is important to become grounded and know more about why you attracted this type of energy. This will become evident as we practice.

Stool pattern: How often do you move your bowels? I evacuate every two to four days.

YC: This is disease causing if not treated.

What is the texture of your stool? Solid and dry.

Does your stool sink or float? It sinks.

YC: This is a sign of heavy or unhealthy digestion.

Is your stool dark or light? Dark.

Does your stool have a strong odor? Yes, sometimes.

Urine: How frequently do you urinate? About 10–15 times a day.

YC: Unless you are drinking a lot, this is quite excessive and will make the skin very dry.

Do you ever urinate during the night (awakening from sleep)? Sometimes.

YC: Avoid drinking any stimulants close to bedtime as they will keep you going to the bathroom.

Does your urine have a strong smell? No, it is light and not very odorous.

YC: This is probably because you drink a lot of water or liquids. Too much water drains the system of good nutrients.

What is the color of your urine? Light yellow.

For women: Menstruation: Do you experience any menstrual pain? I sometimes experience pain in the back or in the legs.

YC: Do a few light postures in a seated position to stretch the lower back and legs.

How many days does your period last? Three to five days.

YC: Good.

Is there much bleeding during your period? There is a little bleeding.

Is your blood dark or light? The blood tends to be light.

YC: Overall, this is a very positive cycle you are experiencing. Little bleeding and light color is fine and healthy for you.

What activities do you engage in during your period? I still exercise, but the workout isn't as strong as I prefer it to be.

YC: This should be a time of rest. Things should be very calm during this time of the month.

Do you experience blood clots during your period? Yes, sometimes.

How would you describe your relationships:

. . . with your friends? I have good friendships, but since I travel frequently for business I only see them about once a month or every other month.

. . . with your partner (if applicable)? N/A

. . . with your parents? I have a great relationship with my parents, though I sometimes struggle with my reaction to some of my father's behaviors.

YC: It is time to let go of the image you have of your father and to move on from this. It will hold you back from your future relationships with men. This will be dealt with during the treatments.

. . . with co-workers? I have a good relationship with co-workers.

. . . with yourself? Generally, it is good. I do sometimes feel overwhelmed by my many thoughts and wind up feeling dissatisfied with who I am.

Other personal comments:

Lately, I've been feeling off balance as I constantly think of many things and feel as though all of my stress is in my head. I do not know how to take control of my thoughts, and I truly think my thinking keeps me from having a relationship or being totally satisfied with myself. There is so much I am grateful for, and there is so much that I have accomplished, and I tend to overlook these qualities.

I believe my history of eating disorders has done a lot of damage to my system, and I am trying to find the right solution to correcting all of this damage. My health is good but not great. My back has improved, but I have been dealing with this for five years and I still have bouts of pain.

At times I tend to have mindless eating moments. I find myself finishing an entire bag of carrots with hummus or a box of crackers and not even realizing what I am doing. I don't even feel full afterward, and I fear that could be an ongoing problem. I want to gain control over this.

YC: To gain control of the mind and therefore to be balanced in your habits, you will need to invest time and effort. You have struggled with these issues and have tried many different ways to change, but it is important for you to realize that it will take patience, discipline, and focus.

Ashtanga: (1) The eight-limbed path outlined by Patanjali in the Yoga Sutras, presenting the necessary steps for a practitioner of yoga to awaken to enlightenment. (2) A fast-paced, aggressive practice of yoga postures taught by Sri K. Pattabhi Jois out of Mysore, India, and throughout the world.

Ayurveda: An ancient system of healing that was created by sages in India over five thousand years ago. Ayurveda calls upon the practitioner to determine the root cause of imbalances in the body and then treat those imbalances accordingly.

Bhagavad Gita: An ancient Hindu scripture outlining the teachings of Lord Krishna as presented to the warrior Arjuna.

Bikram yoga: A modern-day system of twenty-six yoga postures practiced in a room set at over 100 degrees Fahrenheit.

Dosha: A basic constitutional energy type in the body as defined by the system of Ayurveda. The three doshas are Pitta, Kapha, and Vata.

Hatha yoga: An all-encompassing system of yoga postures practiced with the intention of purifying the body for extensive periods of higher meditation.

Kapha: One of the three doshas in the system of Ayurveda. Kapha energy is comprised of the earth and water elements and is responsible for forming our bodies and rooting us.

Kripalu yoga: A modern-day system of yoga postures focusing on gentler sequences.

Kriya yoga: An ancient practice of yoga that makes heavy use of breathing techniques to assist the practitioner in finding self-realization. This practice was made known in the West by Paramahansa Yogananda in his book *Autobiography of a Yogi.*

Pitta: One of the three doshas in the system of Ayurveda. Pitta energy is comprised of the fire and water elements and represents the heat and digestive fire in the body.

Puja: A symbolic ceremony in Hindu and Buddhist traditions that calls upon the practitioner to make an offering to a deity or concept. The deity is a representation of the different energies of the creator.

Sanskrit: An ancient language of India. Many traditional Indian texts such as the Bhagavad Gita and the Yoga Sutras were originally written in Sanskrit.

Vata: One of the three doshas in the system of Ayurveda. Vata energy is comprised of the air and ether elements and is responsible for movement and elimination in the system.

Vinyasa: A modern-day system of yoga postures derived from Ashtanga yoga and popular in Western yoga centers and gyms.

Yoga: An ancient Indian system developed as a tool for eliminating mental afflictions and finding balance in the mind. It is not classified as a religion.

Yoga Sutras: An ancient text authored by the sage Patanjali sometime around the second century BCE. It is considered to be the foundational text of modern yoga.

Yuj: A Sanskrit word that means "yoke" or "to join," as in the joining of the body, mind, and spirit.

Yuga: A cycle as defined by Indian tradition that quantifies humanity's relationship to a collective awakening. Yugas are considered to span hundreds and sometimes thousands of years.

resources

Coelho, Paolo. *The Alchemist.* San Francisco: HarperOne, 1993.

Frawley, David. *Yoga and Ayurveda.* Twin Lakes, WI: Lotus Press, 1999.

Frawley, David, and Vasant Lad. *The Yoga of Herbs.* Twin Lakes, WI: Lotus Press, 1986.

Lad, Vasant. *Ayurveda: The Science of Self-Healing.* Twin Lakes, WI: Lotus Press, 1984.

Mandino, Og. *The Greatest Salesman in the World.* New York: Bantam, 1968.

Rama, Swami. *Living with the Himalayan Masters.* Honesdale, PA: Himalayan Institute Press, 1978.

Seuss, Dr. *The Butter Battle Book.* New York: Random House, 1984.

Tirtha, Swami Sada Shiva. *The Ayurvedic Encyclopedia.* 2nd edition. New York, NY: Sat Yuga Press, 2007.

Yogananda, Paramahansa. *Autobiography of a Yogi.* Los Angeles, CA: Self-Realization Fellowship, 1997.